I0458868

The
Cancer That
Healed Me

ONE WOMAN AND HER JOURNEY
OF FAITH TO NATURAL HEALING

KRISTI WILKINSON

Scripture quotations taken from The Holy Bible, New International Version®, NIV®. Copyright © 1973, 1978, 1984, 2011 by Biblica, Inc. Used with permission of Zondervan. All rights reserved worldwide. www.zondervan.com

Published by Inspire Books
www.inspire-books.com

Cover and Interior Design by Jose Pepito

Print ISBN: 978-1-961065-40-6
e-book ISBN: 978-1-961065-41-3

This book is for general informational purposes only and is not intended to be a substitute for professional medical advice, diagnosis, or treatment. Please consult with your healthcare provider or other qualified health professional regarding any specific health concerns or before undertaking any health-related advice or treatment suggested in this book. The information presented here reflects the author's personal experiences and opinions and should not be relied upon as a substitute for professional medical expertise and is not meant to treat, cure, or prevent cancer or any other disease.

Printed in the United States

Contents

Acknowledgments

First, I want to thank everyone in my family for encouraging me in the choices that I made that were not always popular and at times felt risky but were nonetheless supported. My husband, Tim, was my rock of Gibraltar on a daily basis and never questioned me but lifted me up with his love and prayers. To my mom, a special thanks for the copious meals and shopping excursions made when I was busy to accommodate my special diet requirements. To my dad, for supporting me in the way he always does through love and humor. I thank my son Lukas, who also passionately desired for me to heal in my own way and was gentle in identifying negative patterns in my life that needed to be addressed, in his loving but uncompromising way.

My sister Julie was also adamant about 100 percent compliance with every attempt I made to right my body in mind, body, and spirit. My niece and nephew Tatiana and Damiano were there before, during and after the dark pandemic to encourage me. They also ate Thai food with me that followed my eating plan and helped me to stay the course and not to deviate from this path toward any sweet cravings.

To Erica Viviani and Jerome Stewart, I thank you for all of the podcasts and videos and scientific information you unearthed in everything from broccoli sprouts to Berberine to assist my body to heal—and for keeping my mind focused on the belief that it could.

To the myriads of doctors mentioned in print who guided me toward healing.

I thank Kristen Moriarty for guiding me to a woman who healed of my type of breast cancer naturally and who inspired me to do the same. I also thank Tanya Becker, who was like a cheerleader, also divinely directing me to two men who healed naturally of cancer and who believed that this was possible for me. I thank Gina Derham for believing that I could heal and for helping me to seek balance and stillness along the way.

I thank my pastor, Chris Bernard, for believing that I would be cancer-free and for following up with my care along the way.

To my friend Lana Lemke, for listening to my plight and discovering insights that brought me closer to my goal. I thank Jesse Almanza for guiding me in decisions toward the final steps in my journey, and for your steadfast prayers. To my friend Chrissy Stone, thank you for your faith and your prayers that brought the desires of my heart to pass.

Thanks to Melanie Turner for standing by me at the hospital when my husband was unable to be there for me. To Michelle Rosenblum, I thank you for being like a sister to me through this challenging time and for supporting me and believing that my faith and God would guide me to ultimate healing.

I thank my sister-in-law Debi Thomas, for sending videos and oils and words of encouragement to bring knowledge to me about cancer and natural healing.

To my brother-in-law Russell Bitter, thank you for also listening to me and encouraging me and praying alongside me until God brought the answer we both hoped for.

A special thanks to Dr. Stacy Mulkey, ND, for guiding me in a holistic and multifaceted approach to healing. To Dr. Chris Kaufmann for identifying the main and other root causes of my dis"ease" and guiding me to the proficient Dr. Rothchild, DDS, who did magical dental work that helped my body to begin healing.

Also, to Dr. Jessica Yackley, who, in her last "apprenticeship" before becoming a chiropractor, encouraged me to find the missing piece to my health puzzle and to not surrender what I believed could transpire if I discovered the root cause of my illness. Dr. Jessica, you truly brought me to the finish line in my healing journey.

I profusely thank Rebecca Elrod, who painstakingly delved into my book with a fine-tooth comb to edit my manuscript word by word and sentence by sentence to make it the best it could be, even after losing hours of work several days in a row.

To Beth Lottig, I thank you for believing in me with each book you have published thus far, and for giving guidance for edits, design, and everything in between that made this come to print.

And lastly but most importantly, I thank God, my Creator and my Healer. You spoke words of confidence over me that I could and would heal naturally and that I should write about my story to help others and for you to shine—as you are ultimately the one who deserves the glory.

1

"Why, Mom?"

My son Lukas and I were the last two remaining at the dinner table when he asked me a probing question. "Why do you think you had to go through years of struggle and all the other issues during your cancer battle before you were healed?" I didn't have to think about this for very long because the journey had unearthed so many discoveries along the way. Without much hesitation, I answered, "Lukas, I believe I had to go through so much so that I could try everything possible and research everything I needed to help someone else in their journey. If I had been 'cured' right away, I wouldn't have discovered all the layers involved in my healing process, and if there's one person that I can help, someone who relates to even one aspect of my healing journey, then it will all have been worth it."

He paused before he replied, "That makes sense. I just wish you didn't have to fight it for so long. I'm so relieved you healed and are on the other side now."

Relief was a fitting word for him, and for me. All my family and circle of friends who supported me during my journey could relate to that word. I had been dealing with the "C" word for a little over nine years, and since it is such a daunting and indescribable word, my mind, body, soul, and spirit were relieved to say the least. Perhaps it's hard to even find a word to describe how I felt and how many others must feel when they hear the words, "You are cancer-free!"

My decision to write this book came with many emotions. One was reluctance, possibly based on my nature to be a people pleaser. I didn't want to offend anyone when writing this, coming off as if I knew how to cure cancer or even that that was why I was writing. In my heart of hearts, I didn't want to undermine anyone's cancer journey, the choices they made, the decisions for treatment, options they needed to consider. I have friends who battled cancer who took other paths and were cancer-free. In no way did I want to claim that their choices weren't the best for them. Another emotion was eagerness. I felt eager to share what I had learned in my nearly decade-long battle with this beast of a disease. The next was urgency and necessity. Since I had healed from cancer after a journey that involved both surgery and natural approaches, I felt a responsibility to share what I had learned and share it as quickly as possible. In some ways, though, I needed time to digest all the things I had learned along the way. I felt I needed time to process, as some lessons might come in the months after my healing, but I knew I wanted to help someone like me, someone who was looking for answers to how they could heal.

Again, I cannot emphasize enough that this is not a book about "how to cure cancer." I feel that each person's healing journey is their own. Doctors from Western and Eastern medicine have spent billions of dollars trying to unlock the mystery of this terrible disease. It would be quite presumptuous of me to claim I knew the secret to this mystery. For instance, I learned in my research that blood type cancers, such as leukemia, do not respond to therapies the way that tumor-based cancers do. And since there are more than 200 types of cancer, I do not believe there is just one way to heal this disease. This book is about my healing journey and mine alone. My hope is that, yes, it will help one person find the missing piece of the puzzle to their cancer battle. I want just one more person to find the strength to face this disease with confidence, and hope and belief that they, too, can heal. May this writing be received with acceptance and not resistance, and as a complement to anyone's cancer healing path.

2

Missed Signals

Fall of 1981 had arrived in my suburban town outside of Philadelphia, Pennsylvania, and with it one of my favorite sports—field hockey! Our head coach at Abington High, Kathy Grebe, instructed our freshman team to run a nearly three-mile course every day before practice began, and my friends Sharon Okamoto and Lynn Wachinski, and I didn't hesitate. We sailed down a large, steep hill—used for the best sledding in winter—and kept stride as we entered a wooded park. We skipped over tree roots that riddled the dirt path we were on while maples and elms in tones of tawny reds and rusty oranges shaded us. The difference for me was that I was struggling to breathe and I felt myself begin wheezing, my face noticeably redder than theirs. I was always so determined to keep up with them that I would never mention the fiery feeling in my lungs, nor my difficulty breathing on anything other than a short sprint.

On one particular day, my mom noticed my face was beet red, and when I came to a sideline for a rest, I couldn't disguise my high-pitched rasp from her. She took me to a doctor, and I learned I had exercise-induced asthma, but since it was not severe—or so I told him—he didn't recommend an inhaler. I didn't want to use anything to help me run or exercise since I didn't notice my sister, Julie, or my friends needing anything to help them breathe when they played sports.

That same school year, later in the spring, the "Soph Hop" was advertised on posters hung in the hallway. It was a dance for sophomores, and I thought nothing of it since I was a freshman, but Lonnie, one of the lacrosse players who commonly bumped into me on his way to practice, asked me to the dance. Surprised and flattered, my face turned every shade of red, and although I wasn't interested in dating him, I admired his courage to ask and said yes.

Wearing a white Jessica McClintock cottony crepe-like dress that gathered at the waist with a red sash—to add a splash of color—and short sleeves that fit tightly around my arms, he escorted me onto the dance floor after fastening a white corsage to my dress. We didn't skip a beat and danced to some fast and slow eighties songs from Michael Jackson to Hall and Oates. After spinning around until I was almost dizzy, I felt an itchy feeling on my face. I excused myself to the bathroom, took one look in the mirror, and noticed a red welt on my face next to my nose! Horrified that I might be developing the largest pimple known to man, I took a minute to check all areas near my forehead and cheeks to see if any other craters were brewing. Suddenly, a wave of nausea came over me, accompanied by perspiration near my eyebrows. Blaming it on freshman nerves, I stoically made my way back onto the dance floor, thankful for the dimly lit gymnasium, the distraction of the music, and all the other nervous teens swaying back and forth to a slow song.

Lonnie was nearly the same height as me, five feet, two inches, and we were back on the dance floor, joined in the rhythm. My arms were laced around his shoulders and neck, and I was gazing calmly into his brown eyes when I noticed the welt on my face turn from an itch to a burn. I removed one hand from around his neck to feel the mound on my cheek, and it now seemed gargantuan to my teen perspective; plus, another one had risen on the same side! My stomach was churning in knots, and I feared I might add to my embarrassment by vomiting all over the dance floor. I imagined the custodian illuminating the floor to clean up after me, exposing my pimply face to everyone, including Lonnie.

Not typically one to be a party pooper or to leave a dance so soon after it had begun, I had no choice but to tell Lonnie I had to get home. Upset that I needed to put a sudden and unexpected end to a dance event I knew he'd planned for and anticipated, I felt just as miserable in my heart as I did in my body. He drove me to my home on Susquehanna Street, dropped me off—of course, without a kiss—and no sooner had I arrived than I broke out in hives from head to foot. My mom greeted me at the door, surprised to see I'd come back so soon. She assessed that the suspicious pimples were not dastardly signs of pubescence, but a severe allergic reaction to—we didn't know what. The nausea was mounting, along with a splitting headache, and I wondered why this was happening to me.

The only thing I could think of happened during one of my softball practices while I was on the field with my teammates. A small prop plane flew overhead, releasing a misty haze. Asking what it was, I was told the plane was spraying a chemical to try and combat the gypsy moth epidemic that was wreaking havoc on our city's trees. Never knowing for sure if this was what caused the hives that spotted and speckled my entire being, I had to take oatmeal baths for an entire week since I couldn't take Benadryl due to an adverse reaction to it. A doctor prescribed a medicine to quell the incessant itching and burning that kept me awake most nights. I was a terrible sleeper anyway and was used to lying awake for several hours before dozing off, so this didn't faze me. Since I was too ill to attend school for a week, Lonnie caught wind, understood my plight, and wrote a sweet card wishing me well. Thankfully, our romance came to a halt, and I never had to tell him that I wasn't interested in dating him, and our friendship remained intact.

To my dismay, with my absence from school, I missed the entire year-end review in my math class, but was still required to take a test the day I returned. I absolutely bombed it. Not only did this upset my teacher with her tightly wound bun on her head, but also my tightly wound, perfectionist nature. Since this was my first really bad score in school, my dad said he was going to celebrate my "D" grade. He wanted to help me realize he wasn't asking me to be perfect with my school performance, and hoped I would take the pressure off myself and discover that a terrible grade wasn't the end of the world.

Around this same time, I learned from my mom that her sister Betsy would also frequently develop whole-body hives. She evidently discovered over the years that she had sensitivities to so many foods, she was really limited in what she could eat. If she happened to find a food that didn't cause problems, she would resort to eating it frequently. Oddly, this really didn't work too well for her because, with the increased consumption, she would become allergic to that food too! Since her condition was worsening, her doctor sent her to a clinic in Texas that had an alternative medical floor, as no other doctor could seem to figure out what was causing her allergies. She was put on a food elimination diet, and the tests from this diet revealed that she was allergic to all but two foods—fish and potatoes. While Aunt Betsy was in Texas, my friend Sharon Okamoto and I were in the same biology class with Mr. Bell, and he was teaching us about genetics. We were studying at Sharon's house one night and took a break to have a snack. After biting into an apple, I developed swollen lips, an itchy mouth, and a red ring of small hives around my mouth. Thankfully, it was a mild reaction, but I mentioned to her that my aunt also struggles with hives, and we both exchanged the idea that if my aunt had these similar reactions, perhaps there was a genetic link. Maybe we were both predisposed to having these aggressive reactions to foods/drinks. Actually, as I thought about it, my sister Julie and my parents didn't have any of these allergies or reactions either, nor did any of them wheeze when they exercised.

Again, my mom took me to the doctor, and I was tested for an allergy to apples. We also discovered my mouth would swell with peaches and nectarines, so I was tested for all three fruits, but the doctor concluded I wasn't allergic to any of them. Not wanting to have an itchy and red swollen mouth, I ended up avoiding these fruits for years. I was perplexed by what might be causing this reaction, and that's the only thing I knew to do.

Flashing back to when I was barely three years old, I also remember suffering from severe constipation. I distinctly recall one particular event, sitting on the toilet in a half bath off our kitchen—my abdomen in severe distress—the pain almost unbearable. My little toddler-self struggled with this annoying malady, an embarrassing problem I don't even like mentioning, and I relied heavily on my mom to help me manage. We chalked it up to that childlike fear, feeling that abdominal pain was a cue to avoid visiting the bathroom. Little did I know there was something deeper behind this gut motility issue.

Learning more about Aunt Betsy, my mom informed me she excessively drank a carbonated cola drink, and also had a hankering for sugar. The doctors suspected this could be a link to the development of her allergies. I vowed to Sharon and my family that I wouldn't drink soda from that time on. I was convinced my genetic makeup was similar to Aunt Betsy's, and I feared being allergic to all but fish and potatoes. And speaking of fish, I didn't even really like the way my mom cooked it—deep fried in grease and slathered with ketchup to mask the taste—so this wasn't a food I desired to incorporate in my daily diet. For the next forty years of my life, I kept that promise, save for a few times when soda was the only thing available to drink. Little did I know, this idea of eliminating soda to help prevent future illness was only one of many things I would need to change. My internal radar was alerted to this one sign, but there were many other signals that were missed.

3

✤

Blindsided

A creature of habit, I scheduled my yearly women's check-up with my OB/GYN, Dr. Beaumont, at the end of March, close to my forty-sixth birthday, so I wouldn't forget. Other than a precarious incident ten years prior when that same doctor saved my life after an ovarian cyst ruptured, blowing out my ovarian vein and causing internal bleeding, I always passed all my female preventive tests with flying colors. In addition to examining me, he ordered my routine mammogram, and I thought nothing of it. I would schedule it as soon as I could and check that off my to-do list. Although they never caused me anxiety since my mom didn't have breast cancer, like many women, I think mammograms are rather uncomfortable and remind me of times when my sister or neighbor kids had a tight grip on my arm, causing me to holler uncle to be freed from their grasp. An appointment was available in late April that suited my work schedule, and, after arriving, I changed into a gown in the dressing room and sat in a frigid hallway, waiting for the exam. Due to the temperature and not my nerves, chills ran up and down my arms. Finally, I was greeted by a friendly female who informed me she'd been doing this for years, and I agreeably stood in each position while she repeated, "Inhale and now hold your breath," as she took images from every imaginable angle. She seemed insistent on capturing an image that seemed so close to my ribcage that when the machine clamped down on my soft, fatty breast tissue, I swore it might just pop! Her experience was validated by the ease with which she flipped the machine this way and that and adjusted the arm height while gingerly handling my breasts. I complimented her for making this dreaded appointment so streamlined and efficient. We said our goodbyes, and I went on my merry way. I was confident I would get a phone call from Dr. Beaumont or his secretary telling me my mammogram was clear, and he'd see me next year.

Well, the doctor's assistant called with a very different message. "Mrs. Wilkinson, the mammogram showed calcifications and dense tissue on your right breast that typically aren't cause for concern, but they are indicators that may detect issues in their early stages. Dr. Beaumont would like you to schedule a biopsy just to be certain; this helps us to be thorough."

Knowing my schedule at work was quite busy, I wondered when I would find time. I was also assisting my tenth-grade son through a homeschool charter, and although he attended school four days a week and spent Mondays at home with loads of assignments, I helped him navigate through the work. He has dyslexia and, being his scribe, would read his books out loud to him since many weren't available on tape, or the audio versions were dysfunctional. To say my schedule was overloaded was an understatement, but I figured I needed to get this biopsy on the books, and then I would be set until next year's physical. No one I knew ever had these calcifications, and it was the first time I had heard of them. Since the mammogram was otherwise negative, I wasn't too concerned.

An appointment that fit my schedule wasn't available until the end of May, and the scheduler asking questions about my job discovered I did heavy lifting at work. She said I would need to rest the day or two after, so I scheduled it for a Friday afternoon at 2:00 p.m. That would minimize my time off work after the procedure, and I could still work up until it was time to leave for the appointment. In healthcare, it seems ironic that we don't have much time off to take care of ourselves.

I worked at The Remington Club, a large facility where I was a physical therapist for my beloved elderly patients who lived there either independently, in assisted living, or were there temporarily for therapy in a skilled nursing unit. The day of my biopsy finally arrived, and I ran out after seeing my patients and drove several miles to the Scripps Clinic. I was grateful to say the least that the same tech, Linda, who had just performed my mammogram, was there to guide me through the biopsy. The combination of her expertise and familiarity put me at ease. She explained that the calcifications they noticed were so far back toward my ribcage that if she hadn't had the experience to capture the image she did, the calcifications of concern would have been missed. Linda was gaining my respect with every minute, and I asked if I could see an image of these annoying growths. As I gazed at the report, they seemed to form the shape of a constellation, somewhat like Orion's Belt.

Accompanying her was a nurse who would be guiding the needle into position, and she asked me to climb up onto a long table. Climbing up a step, I lay down on my stomach on a padded mat, and Linda led my breast through a hole in the mat. They both informed me this procedure usually took thirty minutes or less, and once they had me in the right position, it would be completed shortly after. Or so they thought. After placing me in several positions, I was asked to roll over for a second, and I noticed a look of consternation on Linda's face. I asked her if everything was okay, and she responded, "The calcifications are at the most posterior part of your breast, close to your chest wall, and the positions I have tried so far are not sufficient." She had me lie down again, and I am not exaggerating when I say Linda tried twenty-five different positions for over an hour to no avail. With an exasperated tone, she said, "I just can't get your body close enough to the table." Remembering I was lying on a one-to-two-inch padded mat on the table, I asked if it could be removed. Linda replied, "Would you mind if we took it off? You'll be lying directly on the metal, but I am running out of options." The nurse chimed in and said, "If we can't get you in the right position, the doctor will have to do a surgical biopsy."

I hadn't expected this and wanted to avoid surgery if possible, so I agreed to lie on the cold metal slab. My arm was dangling off the table, and my breast was in the hole in the table, but I still was not close enough. Linda had an idea to place both my right arm and breast into the hole so the area could be accessed more easily. They told me they needed to be sure I didn't move, so a device was used to immobilize my neck on the metal table. They commented that they finally had the right position and reiterated that I needed to remain still. I feared that if I told them the pain was building, they would have to call a halt to the entire exam. My physical therapy brain cells were reeling with medical terms, and I didn't want to say a word, but I felt my upper trapezius muscle being compressed, and I feared my plexus of nerves were being compressed as well. The pain was excruciating, and I remember thinking this was the most barbaric procedure I could have imagined. I had to hold still in this position for quite some time as the needle entered, but then they wanted to look at another area and had to remove and reinsert the needle again! Symptoms of lightheadedness were developing due to the extreme pain. I thought to myself, *Not many people would be able to tolerate this pain, and I won't be able to for much longer.* Finally, Linda announced, "We're done. You can sit up now." My first thought was, "Thank God, or I think I would be headed to the surgical biopsy!" I couldn't have tolerated the pain for much longer.

The nurse informed me that Dr. Beaumont would have the results within a week and would call me. I was supposed to perform only light duties over the weekend, and I could return to work Monday. Having mentioned I was lightheaded, they both helped me get off the table. I thanked them for their persistence and asked what time it was. To my surprise, it had taken two and a half hours rather than thirty minutes! Not your typical biopsy, I suppose. I went to the dressing room and looked in a mirror on the way out of the office and noticed a red mark on the side of my neck and upper shoulder girdle where I was being secured by the metal. After the fifteen-minute drive home, the mark was still there. I showed it to my mom, explaining how excruciating it was, and we both noticed it lasted the remainder of the day; it was still a faint, pink line the next morning. My interest was piqued by how women could be screened without having to endure such intense, torturous pain. Knowing that it was for a good reason gave me solace, but still, I hoped other women wouldn't have to bear what I did that day.

I was certain Dr. Beaumont would take at least a week to call me with the results, so I was uncomfortably surprised that very next Monday at work, with Tammy Wadase and Winnie Gelle at my side, when I noticed the Scripps contact number flashing on my phone screen. Alarm bells went off in my head, and even though I typically don't answer calls during the day from telemarketers, or even friends for that matter, I quickly answered the phone. Dr. Beaumont gently said, "Kristi, I have the results of your biopsy. I am so sorry to tell you this. You have breast cancer, but it is DCIS, or ductal carcinoma in situ. It is only stage zero, so the good news is that we caught it early. It has not even developed into a tumor yet. It may sound odd to say this, but if there is cancer to get, this is the best type of cancer to have. There are excellent treatments available, and you will get through this. I will send this information to the Scripps cancer treatment specialists, and they will call you to set up an appointment with the oncologist, plus any following appointments. I will be here if you have any questions, but you are in better hands with the oncologist at this point."

I thanked him for calling so quickly and said that I would keep him informed. His voice was so caring and calming, but I felt like I had been hit by a truck. Cancer? Me? Breast cancer?! This was the furthest thing from my mind! I was so caught off guard that the only thing I knew to do was tell Tammy and Winnie, who both soothed me with a huge embrace as I unexpectedly burst into tears. I do tend to be empathetic, crying at commercials about weak and bony dogs who need foster homes, or movies where a mother's son is on life support, but I didn't like to share tears with friends about my own personal battles. Tammy and Winnie carefully and kindly asked me a little about the phone call without delving too deep, and they assured me they would support me through this process. I still needed to see an entire afternoon of patients and knew I couldn't call Tim, my mom, dad, Julie, or Lukas until I finished work. My mind was fuzzy and fragmented, unable to fully process, let alone digest, the information that had been handed to me. I would need to completely block it out until I got home. The rest of the day was a blur, and thankfully, I was able to treat all my patients, document efficiently, and then drive home to tell my family the news.

4

The Dreaded "C" Word

As I drove home, I was in autopilot, and visions of cancer cells dancing through my body started to overwhelm me. I knew my behavior was overly dramatic, but something about the "C" word does this to a person, at least it did to me. Stage zero, what does that even mean? A song came on the radio that hummed words of hope, but I wasn't able to discern them. Everything was unclear. I arrived at my house—only a seven-minute drive from work—and walked in the door looking for my mom. I knew Tim wouldn't be home from work, and I didn't want to tell Lukas yet as he was a worrier by nature. My mom was in the kitchen, where I often found her, giving me the gift of cooking since I worked full-time and also homeschooled Lukas full-time. I didn't have much more in the tank to cook anything other than a frozen pizza, so she took this task on as her own.

Without hesitating, I said, "Mom, Dr. Beaumont called me with the results, and I have breast cancer." The waves of emotion flooded me again, and those unwelcome tears streamed down my face. After she comforted me with a warm embrace, she responded, "Kristi, I am so sorry. Do you know anything more about it?" This next phrase was one I would retell so many times to friends and family. "Yes, it is stage zero, which I've never even heard of and don't understand yet, but he said that it's in my ducts and that if you're going to get cancer, it is the best kind to get." Whatever that meant about the best kind of cancer to get, I was not sure yet, either, but I would take it for now. I had to stay positive and get out of that mental space where I pictured it multiplying tenfold throughout my body.

My mom then said, "Well, we'll do whatever we need to do to get you through this. I know if it's not even a stage I, you are going to beat this." We both agreed that I would tell Tim next, and then my dad, since he usually was the last one to walk through the door. I would wait until I felt the timing was right to tell Lukas. I wanted to do a little more research before I talked to him about it. No need to scare him unnecessarily.

When Tim came home from work, I could tell he was exhausted from the paint dappled and drizzled all over his clothes, hair, and extremities. As a construction contractor, he was renovating a front deck and performing minor household repairs for my friend, Erica Viviani, and since it was a forty-minute drive in bumper-to-bumper San Diego traffic, I knew he needed a moment to decompress before I hit him with the news. After he showered and dressed, and was about to leave the bedroom, I said, "Hon, I got the news from my biopsy, and I have breast cancer." My attempt to be stoic was a waste, and again, crocodile tears welled up in my eyes and spilled over the rims. As he held me, I noticed tears in his eyes too, dripping down his cheeks onto mine. Now, I said I was typically not a crier when it came to most of my own trials, but I had only seen Tim cry once in our five years of marriage, after his father passed away. I hadn't anticipated this evoking such emotion in him, and I have to say it was truly comforting. Perhaps at times we forget the depth of emotions we have for each other, and his expression of love was soothing to my heart.

My dad arrived home from his job at a golf school in Temecula with his bubbly expression of, "I'm home, what's for dinner?" but he could tell by the look on my face that something was awry. Without him having to ask, I blurted out the news, "I got my results back today from Dr. Beaumont, and

I have breast cancer." He, too, hugged me as he said, "Kristi, I am so sorry." I again went into the explanation that would be repeated again and again to my friends. I wasn't one to keep things like this to myself, like some would. Many people I knew had kept their cancer diagnosis private, not disclosing too much before finding out more, perhaps to protect themselves, and I respected that. I even wondered if that was the better way, but nonetheless, I was the opposite. For me, it was healing to share with my close friends and family members. I had always kept in touch with many friends from high school and college and wanted to let them know what I was going through.

I called Erica, also a physical therapist, and filled her in on the news. After words of solace, she said, "I am going to look into this, and if I can help you in any way, I am here for you, Kristi." She asked, "Have you told Lukas yet?" to which I responded I hadn't but planned to later this evening or the next day. He had a test the next day in history, and I didn't know if the timing was right yet.

That night, as thoughts that I had cancer settled into my soul, I wondered why I ended up getting it. We didn't have a family history of cancer, other than an aunt on my mother's side. She had been a smoker, so I attributed her case to that. I was forty-six, and I felt too young to have cancer, even though I was well aware of many young people and children struck with the disease. Every year, I would join many of my work friends, prompted by my coworker, occupational therapist Belinda Hill, to walk in the Relay for Life, and every year we walked past poster after poster advertising the depressing and rising statistics on women with breast cancer—not to mention the plethora of other cancers. I never imagined I would join that one in eight statistic. I really didn't want to be in that club. But here I was, lying in bed beside my husband, wondering what the next step would be. Would I need chemo or radiation? I was assuming a surgery would be involved. I needed to stop the relentless questions that came in waves, knowing I wouldn't have answers until I saw the oncologist. That day couldn't come soon enough!

After I shut my mind off from the questions, I resolved to tell Lukas after his test the next day. He wasn't a good test taker anyway, with his dyslexia, and I didn't want to give him one more reason to struggle. Finally, I did what I knew in my heart would bring me comfort. I read a devotional before I went to sleep and prayed that God would guide me through this journey called cancer. I didn't want it, didn't ask for it, and truly wanted to believe I had never heard the doctor's words, but I had to face it. Something inside seemed to whisper that it would be ok. I hoped that faint, still voice was right.

5

Strength for My Son

The tears I shed with my friends at work, my mom, dad, and Tim would need to be contained, or at least more controlled, for Lukas. I needed to be strong for him. He wasn't comfortable with medical challenges or my tears and never had been. He'd been riddled with digestive issues since the day I adopted him when he was four-and-a-half, and he tended to be hypochondriacal when it came to ailments from head to toe. If someone he knew had appendicitis, he wondered if he, too, would soon be lying on the operating table, so I felt I needed to handle our conversation with care and strength. Of course, cancer was one of his biggest fears! Even if I didn't yet feel confident about what I was facing, I needed to show him a confident side so he wouldn't worry about me.

After he came home from school, sharing that he felt he did rather well on the multiple choice questions of his exam and was able to recite his answers to essay questions face-to-face with his teachers—one of his accommodations for dyslexia—I decided it was time to talk to him about my diagnosis. I shared with him what I had learned from the doctor: that I had stage zero breast cancer, and since it was not yet a tumor, there was nothing to really worry about. As far as I knew, it hadn't spread anywhere else in my body, and the doctors were confident they could manage it well.

He asked, "Mom, do you think you'll need surgery?" I responded that I didn't know what my options were yet, but I imagined I would. He had a somber expression on his face and was quiet, retreating into his own private thoughts without sharing much. With concern on his face and a furrowed brow, he questioned, "Are you going to be okay?" Managing to keep any tears in check, I replied with conviction, resolve, and a surprisingly soft, assured answer that I knew I would be ok. He may have needed that more than I did. He gave me a hug and held on longer than most teenagers do. He followed with, "Let me know if they want you to have surgery. I want to know." He then walked to his room, and from experience, I knew it best not to talk about it a lot with him, but to share the important details. I wanted more than anything to beat this cancer for him, probably more than for me. Again, I was frustrated that the one disease he feared the most would strike me. I remembered his words as a child regarding Stephanie Cain, my friend who battled metastatic cancer, "Mom, cancer is the devil's disease." His words came to me again strongly after he'd walked down the hall. As I thought about it, that was true in my belief. No disease is from God, but from God's enemy. Some may not ascribe to this way of thinking, but since this is what I believed, I knew I had a battle before me. Now, it was time to win this battle!

6

Consultations Begin

My first of many scheduled appointments was with my new oncologist, and it was a positive one. Dr. Melissa Torrey was five feet tall, possibly less, and she entered the room where I was waiting with my mom with the confidence and enthusiasm to match the height of her shiny black heels. I felt assured almost before she opened her mouth. After introducing herself, she explained, just as Dr. Beaumont had, that DCIS or ductal carcinoma in situ was very curable since it was considered a stage zero, slow-growing, and non-aggressive type of cancer. She also described that it was HER2 negative, but hormone receptor-positive, which she explained meant first that the breast cancer cells didn't have abnormal levels of HER2 proteins, but were fed by estrogen and could benefit from a medicine that would inhibit or suppress the estrogens in my body and breasts.

Next came her recommendations, which were straightforward and based on her research. Being a biology major in college, I appreciated her candid nature, which was clinically driven. She recommended I have a lumpectomy and not a mastectomy. A mastectomy would be too aggressive in her scientific opinion, because stage zero meant that, although malignant, it hadn't formed into a tumor yet. She also stated she wasn't recommending chemotherapy, nor did she recommend radiation at this time. She suggested I keep radiation in my "back pocket" as a targeted approach if the cancer were to recur. The recurrence rate was less than 15 percent with or without radiation after a lumpectomy, and although she would follow my care, my chances were high that she most likely would not have to recommend any aggressive interventions. In conclusion, she approached the topic of a medication, Tamoxifen, that she would circle back to after my surgery. Apparently, it acts as a suppressant she sometimes prescribes for a five-year minimum to suppress the estrogens that may influence a recurrence. Admitting that this was a lot of information, she asked what my reactions were to everything she said. She asked if I had any initial inclinations toward treatment approaches, stating that if I needed time to delve into this further, she was not rushing me, nor did I have to make any immediate decisions. Expressing that I would go forward with the lumpectomy, I had already agreed that a mastectomy would be too aggressive, as I didn't tend to make decisions based on the fear of what could be. As of this writing, I learned from a friend going through the same type of cancer as mine that insurance no longer pays for mastectomies for stage zero breast cancer, as they don't deem it necessary. I also expressed that I was thankful chemotherapy was not part of the treatment protocol, and I was leaning toward her suggestion about leaving radiation as a future weapon. Radiation was something I decided to further research on my own, and as my consultation ended, she explained that the cancer team nurse would be scheduling an appointment with the surgeon and the radiation specialist, and I didn't have to rush into any decisions. She infused assurance in me that, with the arsenal of treatment methods available, I would have a positive outcome nonetheless. I have to admit I couldn't have been matched with a more perfect oncologist, and I let her know I would follow up with her after my surgery. Her positive outlook, her caring nature, her conviction about the future looking bright and cancer-free made my worries wane and my hopes soar as I left the office with my mom. To this day, I am thankful I took every bit of her advice.

Shortly after meeting with Dr. Torrey, the triage nurse booked an appointment with Dr. Pamela Kurtzhals, who came highly recommended by my work friend, Belinda Hill. This appointment was likewise uplifting and met with assurance, hearing about her years of expertise as a breast specialist. She had humor that was not ill-received, but rather welcomed to ease the tension for a surgery of such gravity. During that initial consult, she did a physical examination and proclaimed, "Your breasts are quite pendulous!" to which I could only chuckle, amused by her word choice. I'm not sure if it was a compliment or a criticism, but I was impressed by her vocabulary since many didn't use this word in common speech. It was an outpatient procedure, and she recommended two weeks of recovery time away from work, which she joked may be a blessing in disguise. It certainly was for me, since I had a habit of overworking. Coming away from her office, I felt I could finally come up for air, breathe deeply, and certainly overcome this quickly.

Dr. Torrey suggested I meet with the radiologist just to be informed in case I decided I wanted radiation treatments right away. Since I had treated cancer patients who had radiation burns and blisters, I was not jumping at this option, but I agreed to meet with the team nonetheless. Tim and I were to meet with the radiologist in the clinic near Torrey Pines, close to the coast, and the building was reminiscent of a Frank Lloyd Wright design, which had organic lines and shapes that seemed in harmony with the nearby shoreline. When we walked in, however, I had a daunting feeling wash over me. The lines were so stark. It felt cold, with only one hard-to-find contact person in a two-story, open concept space. Sparse to few patrons sat in the waiting area staring blankly, seemingly having had every emotion but fear sucked from them. Instantly, I didn't resonate with this area or this idea, but decided I would remain open to the expertise of the doctor. Tim and I waited for quite some time before a male doctor greeted us and rapidly spewed out fact upon fact about radiation, drawing mathematical graphs followed by percentages in a very matter-of-fact way. Scribbled circles and lines drawn on a very small piece of paper were meaningful to him, but were delivered in such a way that the information went everywhere and nowhere all at once. I am a science girl, left-brained for sure, but I understood almost nothing he said. Tim asked a few pointed questions that were helpful since I was almost speechless, and then the doctor asked me about my alcohol consumption, to which I responded that I drank fewer than six glasses of wine a year. Tim chimed in jokingly that he usually finished half of the six glasses for me, so my count was half off. The doctor, unamused, stated blandly that this was an acceptable amount to drink, and then encouraged us to consider radiation and everything else he'd mentioned. He did, however, concur with my oncologist that it could be kept as an option for later if I developed cancer again.

Since I trusted Dr. Torrey, I opted for surgery only, meaning I didn't have to decipher the statistics and numbers scribbled on that tiny piece of paper. Whew! I hoped this would be the last time I had to go to that stale, cold, lifeless building with stark angles to match.

There was only one more visit with an oncology nurse who was very knowledgeable and came highly recommended. This was the last of the appointments, and since my friend Belinda spoke so highly of her, I was actually looking forward to meeting her. She was a seasoned woman, with salt and pepper hair and a cut that matched her professional nature. During this appointment, I learned that fried foods, red meat, and alcohol were on the avoid list, and since I didn't eat or drink much in that vein, I thought the diet suggestions wouldn't be challenging. This nurse would follow me after the surgery and every six months until I was in the clear. Belinda was right. She was bright, confident, encouraging, and filled with years of experience, so I walked away mustering energy and positivity for the road ahead. I walked forward blindly, armed with the instructions of the medical practitioners. I didn't have many questions, but those would begin in the blink of an eye.

7

D-Day

Since the 2008 crash in the economy, Tim had taken on work in Northern California, about ten hours away, and he only traveled home once a month to be with Lukas and me. Of course, for this, he made an exception! He went to as many appointments with me as he could, and made certain he'd be there for me on the day of my surgery. The night before, as we lay next to one another, he reached for my hand and we prayed together that the doctor's hands would be guided to a successful outcome. Tears streamed down both of our cheeks as he held me close. I hadn't anticipated cancer as a part of my life, yet I was thankful to have such support. It allowed me to see a vulnerability in him that I didn't often see. A caregiver by nature, this reversed the roles and allowed me to be on the receiving end of the same devotion he'd shown his father when I met them both at my rehab facility, the very same support that touched me deeply and attracted me to him. With Tim by my side, a sense of peace came over me and invited me to a restful sleep, something that typically eluded me.

I was scheduled for the first surgery of the morning, and thankfully, close to our home in Poway, I checked in at the Scripps Clinic at 7:00 a.m. A lumpectomy was planned, and after Tim hugged me—an embrace that assured me everything would be fine—I was ushered into the pre-op room and handed a piece of paper. Looking at it, I was sure someone had made a mistake. At the top of the page, just below my full name, was the surgical procedure I awaited—partial mastectomy. What?! With a lump in my throat, anxiety filled every cell in my body, and I could barely breathe. I thought to myself, *I need to talk to the surgeon before I get whisked back into surgery to make sure she isn't cutting off half of my breast*! With the weight of an elephant on my chest, I mustered up the courage to speak to the nurse who'd handed me the paper and asked, "I'm having a lumpectomy and not a partial mastectomy, right?" She quelled my overwhelming fear and said, "Don't worry, that is a coding thing. We have to code it and write it that way so the insurance company will reimburse us correctly. If we only write lumpectomy, we won't get adequately reimbursed." *Phew*!! I thought to myself. My lungs decided they could breathe again, and my blood pressure—bound to have risen a few points—returned to its happy place. Since I work in healthcare, I knew the importance of coding medical procedures and diagnoses accurately, and, even if 'partial mastectomy' was a half-truth, I was thankful for any financial savings this would afford me. No more questions. I was ready.

After being rolled to the operating room, Dr. Pamela gave me a warm greeting and said we were almost ready to roll. I briefly met the anesthesiologist who mentioned I would be asleep before I could count to ten, and as he injected medicine into the port the nurse had prepared for him, I barely got to the number four before I was in never never land.

The surgery was complete, and voices swirled around me, but I didn't have the ability to respond quite yet. As I lay limply on the table, I realized I could hear clog-clad feet tapping busily across the floor and conversations floating around me, but my eyes wouldn't open and my mouth couldn't form words. Finally, one nurse, wondering when her sleeping beauty would "come to," eagerly asked me if I was ready to get up. Uttering my first words, I said I was alert but unable to move my body. Evidently, I had been in recovery for hours, far longer than anyone expected. They'd informed Tim I might be awake and ready to leave by 9:30 a.m., and here it was, already noon! I told the nurse that as soon as my paralyzed state subsided, I would be ready to go. As I was rousing, I was given discharge instructions and told I had been fitted with a harness-type bra that I was to wear for the next two weeks, 24/7, save for shower time. As I became more mentally aware, I realized "harness" was more like an upper-body straightjacket, but Dr. Kurtzhals insisted on its use to preserve my shape, so I promised 100 percent compliance. When my extremities finally came to life like a marionette dangling from strings, and after being hoisted into a wheelchair with the aid of a male nurse, I was finally reunited with Tim, and we made our way home.

I was informed during discharge that I wasn't to shower until the next day, so as I prepared to unfasten my breast harness twenty-four hours later, there was a significant level of trepidation. I really needed help from Tim, but part of me wanted to witness my breast for the first time on my own. Tim unfastened the clasp for me, but I told him I wanted to be alone as I removed the harness and bandages in the shower. I wondered to myself if I would look disfigured and, since the insurance claim said I needed a partial mastectomy, would the surgeon need to take an extra scoop of tissue to pacify the billing department? Hesitating for a moment, I gingerly removed the bandages, and to my amazement and surprise, I could barely notice any change at all in my breast shape! The cancer cells migrated so close to the side of my body and my ribcage that my breast was nearly unscathed, other than by the incision line. Dr. Kurzhals was a GENIUS, and I decided then and there to completely dismiss her jocular comment about my breasts succumbing to gravity. I excitedly called for Tim to come back into the bathroom, showing him her surgical handiwork, and we both marveled at her expertise. This was not nearly as awful as I had anticipated, and I was so thankful for the advancements in this field, which attempted—as much as possible—to keep a woman's body intact, despite the disease.

As I showered, tears of relief fell from my cheeks, melding with the warm water streaming down my body. I thought to myself, *I am on the other side now*, hoping I wouldn't have to go down this path again.

8

Take Me Away to Telluride

With a post-op visit two days after surgery, and having two weeks off in the middle of August, I impulsively planned a weeklong vacation with Tim to join Lukas and my parents at Julie's home in Telluride, Colorado. A thirteen-hour drive ahead of us, we pulled away from the house Thursday morning, just three days after Monday's surgery. Of course, I didn't ask any of the doctors about traveling so soon after surgery, especially to a 9,000-foot elevation. Tim thought we should wait a few more days, but I was eager to get to the majesty of the mountains and the crisp, clean air. I assured him I would be fine.

No sooner did we get to the Flagstaff, Arizona, area than my head began to pound. Had I forgotten the reality of mountainous elevations and their effect on able-bodied travelers, or had I just been too headstrong, wanting to get there to soak up every moment I could in this area I loved? As we climbed higher and higher, the head pain intensified accordingly. I became nauseated and questioned whether to tell Tim, because—UGH—I would be admitting I was wrong. Even so, I pushed my pride into the backseat and revealed my plight. There was not a doubt in my mind that we should have waited, as he suggested, but there was no turning back. Surrounded by the gold and reddish hues of the Painted

Desert, we made our way through the Native American towns of Tuba City and Kayenta.

Suddenly, it seemed all the moisture was just sucked out of my head, like the arid land around me. I thought I might hurl on the side of the road as we meandered through the mountain towns of Dolores and Rico, and drove over Lizard Head Pass, but I kept my eyes closed and my breathing slow and rhythmic, in concert with the pulsing of my head. Tim was my guardian angel, turning off the music and kindly refraining from conversation, knowing how miserable I was. He forged ahead, only stopping to get me more water. We finally arrived at Julie's house in Placerville, just thirty minutes outside Telluride and at 8,500 feet, and the beauty of it all settled my spirits, family warmed my soul, and the hugs from Julie, her husband Nicola, and her kids Tatiana and Damiano left me assured that this would be a healing place. My head pain had not lessened one bit, but my heart was exploding with joy.

After re-hydrating and getting a good night's rest, my headache thankfully lessened to a mild nuisance, and I was ready to absorb the magic of my surroundings. Towering in front of Julie's home, the peaks of Mt. Wilson were laced with Aspen trees that danced and twinkled like hummingbird wings and seemed to sing to me. They silenced my fears and quieted my soul, and I knew this was just the place I needed to rest and restore, bra-harness or not.

The oncology nurse told me she would be calling me within a week to let me know the results of the biopsy taken during surgery. Since my cancer was stage zero, in my heart of hearts, I wasn't worried about it. Honestly, I expected everything to be behind me. I awaited her phone call with anticipation, perhaps an ounce of hesitation, believing I would get the "all clear" message when I heard from her. It was a Saturday. Alone, I went for a short walk, ironically surrounded by the same astounding beauty featured on my job's screen saver in California. Oddly, this wasn't by design; just some photographer who wanted to share this incredible scenery with other people around the globe. Only a mild ache reminded me of what I believed was behind me, and the crisp mountain air rejuvenated me. Returning to the house, Tatiana and Damiano, and some of their friends were excited to see the latest "Despicable Me" movie with those surprisingly endearing, dome-shaped minion characters. Knowing Julie had many things to coordinate to have all of us at her home, I eagerly offered to take them.

Then the phone rang. I noticed the number was from Scripps Hospital and knew this was not a great sign. Unless something is urgent, positive results are typically shared during the business week. Instantly, a feeling of anxiety washed over me. My oncology nurse was on the other end of the phone and said, "Although the surgery went well, the margins are not clear. There are two areas at ten o'clock and two o'clock that tested positive for cancerous cells, and the surgeon will need to do a repeat lumpectomy. I suggest you do this as soon as possible, as she can most likely use the incision line from the first surgery, and since you will be off work for an additional two weeks, you can apply for short-term disability. I can start that paperwork for you. Do you have any questions?"

QUESTIONS? I was speechless! My mind couldn't think, I couldn't process. I was so certain the surgeon would have gotten all the cancer cells the first go-round! Completely deflated, I put on a brave face and told Tim, my parents, and Julie that I would need to call on Monday, get the procedure scheduled, and prepare for surgery number two to remove the invasive cells still lurking in my breast. As it was time to leave for the movie, I gathered the kids and their friends, and we drove up the neighboring hillside into Telluride. Quietly, I sat down in the theater. The advertisements ended, and the film began. In the darkness that shrouded my face from onlookers, the gravity of the situation fell upon me, and the tears followed suit. I had to rein in my emotions from the kids, as I didn't want my sadness to be interpreted as fear. Of course, this time, the surgeon would get the cancerous cells in the mysterious margins, but I honestly just didn't want her to have to cut me open again and deal with the pain and the assault on my body. After mentally checking out for at least a third of the movie, I pulled myself together. A flood of tears had pooled above my upper lip, and I wiped them off with the long-sleeved T-shirt I'd carried along for the chill of the air-conditioned theater, deciding to lose myself in those little goggle-eyed minions that reminded me of the Weebles I collected in the seventies. My sadness was satisfactorily hidden from my small tribe of kids, whose laughter brought me to a happier place. I would push the thoughts and emotions aside and buckle up for the next step.

Later, a few comments about natural healing started swirling in my head, the ones that had come from my mom and sister, and some of my coworkers back in San Diego. I decided that when I returned home, and after the next surgery, I would use my time away from work researching some of the ideas they mentioned. For now, I needed to enjoy the remainder of my trip and the majesty surrounding me.

9

D-Day 2.0

After only partially digesting the news that I would need an additional surgery, I called Scripps on Monday and uneventfully scheduled it exactly two weeks after the first one. I navigated through the disability paperwork without a glitch, and would have a total of four weeks off from work, which, honestly, was a welcomed break. Since we were dealing with the same surgical site, Dr. Kurtzhals didn't need to meet with me again, thankfully. One less appointment to manage.

The day arrived. Since Tim had needed to return to work, my close friend, Melanie Turner, offered to take me to my appointment, and, after picking me up at my house, we first stopped at Torrey Pines, on the coast, and Melanie prayed with me. When we arrived at the hospital, a refreshing and beautiful coastal breeze welcomed us. To have the comfort of this friend who had also been with me in the hospital after having a C-section for twins was just what I needed; a calming presence and not one to bring more drama to the situation. Melanie stayed and waited with my mom, who arrived later to take me home. When the anesthesiologist approached me before surgery, I was quick to inform him I felt overly sedated after the previous procedure, and he assured me he would make the necessary adjustments. Dr. Kurtzhals encouraged me before I went back to the surgical suite, saying this time, she would get everything. Afterward, she let my mom and Melanie know everything had gone smoothly and she would see me for a follow-up appointment in a few weeks.

Since I'd known what to expect, this surgery had, in a sense, been uneventful. Dr. Kurtzhals kept her word, following the same incision line and taking barely any noticeable tissue since I was still stage zero and only cells, rather than a tumor, needed to be removed. She told me she hoped we wouldn't need to see each other again, and I was more than pleased with her work and thankful to be over this hurdle. Or so I thought.

At home, I stuck to that promise I made to myself and made plans to investigate cancer and the suggestions people had given me about natural healing. To me, "back in the day," daytime TV was so dreadful, with soap operas or game shows as the only choices for entertainment. Once the two days of Vicodin pills were no longer needed for pain, I was ready to get going on my reading. Speaking for myself, I can barely form sentences on narcotics, let alone read or concentrate. During my recuperation, I was pleasantly surprised by visits from my friends and coworkers Winnie Gelle, Marie Graber, and Tammy Wadase, who brought with them flowers and well wishes for a smooth recovery. Touched by their gesture of kindness, I was motivated for the two-week study to begin.

10

Mad Scientist?

My ninth-grade biology class with Mr. Bell birthed in me a love of science that exists to this day. Once he detailed the miracle of genetics and DNA, I knew I was hooked! I majored in biology in college and pondered the thought of becoming a coroner until my first exposure to an autopsy during my senior year, when I inhaled. Picturing myself as a modern-day Columbo, a disheveled but brilliant detective popular on a TV show in the seventies, my AP biology class headed to downtown Philadelphia, to the morgue. My science class friends, Duane Sewell, Sharon Okamoto, and I circled around the coroner as he made an incision on a corpse, commenting that the person had been a heavy drinker, which explained his overly odiferous state. It was as if the fumes coming from his body had the power to push me right out the door and onto a new career path! Even so, that internal instinct to investigate and research still resounds in me today.

Just after my initial cancer diagnosis and before my first surgery, a lovely coworker named Shareen—born in Kenya, Africa, and having moved to the US at a young age—gently asked if I would mind her sharing some information about cancer with me. She must have known this was a sensitive subject, one that not everyone invites suggestions. But I was somewhat new to my cancer journey, and I welcomed her knowledge. She mentioned that someone in her family had battled cancer, and there was a doctor named Gerson who treated cancer naturally and wrote a book about it. With high hopes, she wanted me to look into getting the book, which swiftly arrived at my door in time for my research to begin. Additionally, a nurse named Phyllis, from the island of Trinidad, interjected that I should avoid multiple biopsies. Apparently, when the body part with cancer is pierced with the biopsy needle, it can cause the cancer to spread. She also mentioned, "Pay attention to your diet. It is very important if you have cancer."

Healing naturally? Diet? These were foreign concepts to me in regard to cancer. My only understanding up to this point was that we didn't contribute to cancer unless we were smoking or inhaling toxic chemicals all day. The teachings I listened to implied we did nothing to cause it; the cancer just appeared in us, and we were at its mercy, with the only options for treatment being surgery, radiation, and chemotherapy. Perhaps these women who approached me so gently but confidently, from countries outside our borders, knew something I didn't. I was ready to explore.

Days before my first lumpectomy and my short leave of absence from work, I received a phone call from my sister-in-law and dear friend, Debi Thomas. Thankfully, in the middle of a lunch break from my current PT position at Casa de las Campanas in Rancho Bernardo, I was able to step outside to speak with her. She stated hesitantly, "Hey, I just watched some videos on cancer, and they were so informative. Do you mind if I tell you a little bit about them?" I let her know I was open to anyone's insight to guide me through this battle. She said, "The video series is called *The Truth about Cancer*. There are approximately eight to ten segments, and it takes a while to complete, but it talks about so many things I wasn't aware of, links they are making to cancer, and suggestions about diet. It's available online, and I think it would be worth your time." I was so thankful she'd watched all those videos, thinking of me, and wanting to share what she'd learned. Of course, I thanked her, knowing that with everything coming up, I'd have to keep them on the back burner. My surgery was already scheduled, and I worked every day up until then, but I wondered and hoped the information Debi shared with me would be helpful.

Now that I had a total of four weeks off and wanted this cancer to be behind me, my research began. I devoured the 410 pages of the book my coworker Shareen suggested, and took notes as I read. It's called *The Gerson Therapy: The Proven Nutritional Program for Cancer and Other Illnesses*, written by Charlotte Gerson, the daughter of Dr. Max Gerson, and Morton Walker, DPM. Max was a German/Jewish doctor who attended the universities of Breslau, Wuerzburg, Berlin, and Freiburg in the early 1900s and happened upon his curative findings for cancer and other diseases by default—his own. While in medical school, he suffered debilitating migraines, and no doctor he consulted could offer him relief. Searching for a cure, he found an article in an Italian medical journal describing a woman who had relieved her migraine symptoms with dietary changes, so he also attempted a dietary approach. After drinking only milk for several days with no improvement, he then resorted to eating only apples, and his symptoms disappeared. In short, many of his patients who also suffered from migraines tried his approach—including the elimination of salt from the diet—and, unbelievably, in addition to the migraines subsiding, other ailments such as tuberculosis of the skin also disappeared. Since he'd been taught tuberculosis was incurable, he was unconvinced and involved himself in the research of 450 patients with this skin ailment, 446 of whom were able to alleviate their symptoms using the diet approach. News spread to Nobel Peace Prize winner Albert Schweitzer, whose wife suffered from lung tuberculosis, and utilizing the same technique, her symptoms also disappeared. Dr. Max Gerson deduced that he was not only treating symptoms, as is the orthodox medical method of treatment, but he was assisting the body in helping itself, using diet as his design.[1]

This resonated with me. Since I had suffered from allergies my entire life, and headaches/stomach aches throughout my adult life, I noticed a repeating theme after consulting with a naturopathic doctor near Boulder, Colorado and later, in California, with a brilliant physician in La Jolla named Dr. Moss. I had been complaining to my longtime friend and fellow physical therapist, Susie Lefebvre, about my unrelenting headaches, and she suggested I see a naturopath in her area. I drove from Denver to Boulder to see him, and he asked what seemed like a hundred questions about my symptoms, eating habits, and my bowel regularity or lack thereof. Interesting that he asked about my bowels, as this had been a lifelong problem for me. After he analyzed my answers, he suggested I avoid eating gluten for one week and determine how I felt. Actually, my headache symptoms disappeared after four days—the time needed, he explained, for the motility of the gut to expel the food eaten—and, informing him of this, told him I didn't feel I needed a repeat visit.

Later in life, after I moved to San Diego, I had six sinus infections within the first six months of living there, and another one of my PT friends, Erica Viviani, introduced me to Dr. Moss, who used to be a physician with a large, traditional hospital. He explained that he left his practice and branched out on his own, as he felt the medical group he worked with wasn't using science to treat their patients. The issue of slow bowel motility, or constipation, a recurring theme, was illuminated, and he explained that if we didn't eliminate stool daily, toxins built up in our colons and contributed to headaches and other bodily aches and pains. He blamed the foods we ate for slowing down our bowels and causing these issues.

Also during my appointment, he tested me for not only my IgG

---

[1] Charlotte Gerson and Morton Walker, *The Gerson Therapy: The Proven Nutritional Program for Cancer and Other Illnesses* (New York: Kensington, 2001), 27.

response, which had a response of anaphylaxis, but also four main hitters—my IgA, IgD, IgE, and IgM. My primary care doctors had simply told me I was not allergic to wheat/gluten, but Dr. Moss tested me with a needle—similar to my mainstream allergist's technique—and, using this different approach, the resulting red rash extended down my entire arm, probably over twelve inches in length. He said a quarter-sized rash would have confirmed a positive, but my reaction was the strongest he'd ever seen. He also tested additional foods, and I had similar rash reactions. His testing even detected allergies to every tree in the surrounding area. He asked me to report back to him after eliminating gluten and four other foods he considered to be the top five allergens: corn, milk, peanuts, and soy. Then, the final blow—he detected a sensitivity to chocolate. *Chocolate?!! NOT CHOCOLATE*, I thought to myself! It was going to be challenging enough to give up those five foods—save for the soy sauce and soy milk, which I had given up years before, thanks to Erika. Now I have to give up chocolate?! I don't think he or I knew how incredibly hard that was going to be, since chocolate and I had developed a love affair after the doctor in Boulder told me to stop eating gluten products. Since I was committed to feeling healthier and avoiding those recurrent sinus infections, I would be diligent in adhering to his recommendations.

A tincture of sublingual drops was created for me to address the plethora of tree-based allergies and dietary restrictions. Since I had already eliminated gluten from my diet for many months in the past, with great results, I was on board with avoiding these new food groups. My headaches disappeared, as did my stomach aches and frequent sinus infections. On one of my follow-up appointments, I remember him saying, "Many of my clients' parents are trying to figure out why their kids get sinus infections, need tubes in their ears, and have bad allergies. Western medicine teaches us that if they don't have an IgG or an anaphylactic reaction, these children are fine with these foods. I believe we need to test for sensitivities as well. Most kids wouldn't need tubes in their ears or inhalers for asthma if parents determined and eliminated the foods to which they were sensitive. Many families just won't make the effort. I hope we see a shift in this." Despite the upcoming flu season, I was not sick again for over a year. I was overwhelmed with the similar theme I was reading in Max Gerson's findings, which equated to, "Change the way you eat, and you can heal thyself."

My visit to the doctor in Boulder was in the 1990s, and to Dr. Moss in the early 2000s. This was well before the "gluten and lactose-free" wave. I believe so many people now are discovering how their symptoms are related to what they ingest. The saying, "We are what we eat," must have some merit after all! I dove even deeper into this Gerson methodology and gathered nuggets that resonated with me. The main tenets of the book suggest eliminating salt and sodium, supplement with potassium, eat tons of leafy greens and all vegetables and raw fruits, use lots of carrot and green vegetable juices to address toxicity and vitamin and mineral deficiencies, limit meat but eat oatmeal, and employ a new and not-so-pleasant approach I'd never heard of or dreamed of—coffee enemas.[2] Yes, I did say coffee enemas! I believe Shareen wisely left out this little gem when telling me about Dr. Gerson's book. Had she introduced me to his theory with enemas in mind, no less using coffee, I would have run the other way. But I was intrigued and learned that these had been used for years, if not millennia! Researchers showed that the use of enemas began 2,000 years ago for the purpose of healing and detoxification, and was even recorded in part of a document in the Dead Sea Scrolls. However, the use of coffee enemas was really only introduced to the public around the time of World War I.[3] Although controversial, debated, and debunked by many in the medical field, I figured if it was working for fifty-plus testimonials

---

[2] Gerson and Walker, *Gerson Therapy*, 35.

[3] Gerson and Walker, *Gerson Therapy*, 156–157.

of people with cancer, arthritis, migraines, and other diseases Gerson listed in his book, why not for me also?

A related side story about oatmeal—since, oddly, my body really didn't get along with this grain, usually touted for all its health benefits—includes a recipe for homemade granola from my friend Sharon Leilich Hollis. At the time, I was being consistent in avoiding gluten, but we had a guest in town, Bill Kaliden. He was one of my dad's best friends from his youth in Pittsburgh, and I knew he enjoyed healthy eating options, so I found my friend's granola recipe and doubled the batch. Not in tune with a recommended serving size of less than half a cup, I poured myself a not-so-modest bowl of granola to enjoy with Bill. Since I was depriving myself of so many gluten treats, couldn't I indulge in a benign bowl of grains and fruit? Within several hours of enjoying this tasty treat, I had a splitting headache, so severe that it incapacitated me from most of my activities. I didn't let on its intensity to Bill or anyone else, but the memory of it haunts me to this day. It lasted two days, which was abnormal for me, but led me to more research, finding that certain oats were also in the gluten family. Aha!—that was the culprit. With the current wave of gluten-free products today, there is gluten-free oatmeal, but I tend to steer away from even this, lest I suffer the possible consequences of a beastly head-pounding ache.

Back to coffee enemas: Gerson believed the cause of most chronic illnesses was toxicity and deficiency of nutrients. He was successful in addressing the issue of deficiency with juicing, but the toxins already in our cells and organs—years of polluted air, water, chemicals in foods, and viruses and germs—released waste products into the bloodstream and on to the liver, overwhelming it and making it too burdensome to release the toxins. The coffee enema was a way to open the bile ducts to allow the liver to release the unwanted toxins.[4] An Austrian doctor—along with other researchers interested in Gerson's work—found that coffee has palmitic

---

[4] Gerson and Walker, *Gerson Therapy*, 30–31.

acid in it, which heightens the effects of certain enzymes that then assist in releasing free radicals from the body.[5] To me, the science behind coffee enemas was incredible, and Gerson's idea of using nutrients to restore the cells made total sense. I became a believer, realizing I might need to keep some of these ideas to myself, especially refraining from sharing my "mad scientist" approach with my oncologist. I felt Shareen shared this information with me for a reason. Those health signals I had throughout my youth—allergies and recurrent illness—had been there all along. I just needed to figure out how to restore my body, and Gerson was going to help me do just that. I determined I wasn't simply a "mad scientist," I was a scientist who was MAD at components of the medical model for only providing one method of healing: prescriptions and surgeries. I was convinced there was more we could do to heal our bodies from within.

---

[5] Gerson and Walker, *Gerson Therapy*, 31–32.

11

The Truth About Cancer

Next in my research itinerary was the video series my sister-in-law Debi Thomas recommended to me, *The Truth about Cancer*. Since I still had time off during my four-week medical leave, I committed to watching the nearly ten-part video series, each at about an hour. Now, I know there's a danger in trying to self-diagnose or apply research about one case to all people. Since there are more than 200 types of cancer—and most likely variants among those types—I found this series to be applicable to myself and most. Although I took notes at the time, sadly, I cannot find them since it was over ten years ago. However, I can summarize some of the videos that struck me. First, I was struck by the information that cancer feeds on sugar. How did I not know this?! This, I found out, was discovered in the 1960s, so why on earth was that not in cancer 101 instruction manuals at every oncology doctor's office? I was actually angered by this. A memory triggered for me when I took my neighbor to a chemotherapy infusion for multiple myeloma, and the staff was offering cookies, candy, and other saccharine treats to their patients. I was horrified! Why, if the doctors knew that cancer fed on sugar, would they be trying to kill the cancer cells with chemo, while pacifying their patients with the parasitic enemy that fed the cancer? Truly, I was speechless.

Whichever teaching module this was in was priceless to me, and I knew I would need to heed its instruction.

Next, I recall a series on mercury amalgam fillings in our teeth and their link to cancer. This is also frequently debated, with some thinking the mercury is fine and others who don't. What I recall most specifically is that dentists were finding links between patients with breast cancer and mercury fillings. Evidently, the mercury could leech out of one's teeth into the bloodstream and become toxic. I find it interesting that the dental industry doesn't share this, but most are ironically no longer using mercury fillings. Many women will agree with me that when visiting one's OB/GYN during pregnancy, warnings are given not to ingest much tuna due to the possibility of mercury toxicity. At least I was warned. I was so convinced, I scheduled an appointment with my dentist to remove all of my mercury fillings. If there was a link for anyone out there, I didn't want it to be me. Little did I know how important a part my teeth would play in my cancer puzzle.

There was also a series on spices, turmeric in particular. It mentioned that cancer statistically is lower in India, where people ingest much more turmeric than Americans, and the research supported this magical spice being known to impair cancer cells. While I was on my medical leave, I had a lot of extra time on my hands, and I love walking outdoors. Out in the cul-de-sac, in front of my house, I encountered my neighbors Nittin and Etka Jain. Since they were from India, I shared my most recent findings on turmeric and cancer. Being an open-book kind of girl, I told them why I was on "vacation," and they were supportive and concerned. Within a few days, there was a knock on my door, and there stood Nittin and Etka holding what must have been a ten-pound bag of turmeric! This was a spice worth the cost of gold to many, and to me it was priceless. I had shared with the Jains that a young, lovely, and highly intelligent doctor at my work, Dr. Hanrahan, had informed me the dosage of turmeric for treating cancer would need to greatly exceed the typical usage in a bowl of chili, so to speak, so they took her at her word and gave me a lifetime supply. I still use it in my vegetable soups and spicy dishes to this day. Maybe there's an expiration date on there somewhere, but their gesture of love and care most certainly extended its shelf life.

I had a good working rapport with Dr. Hanrahan, and since she knew about my cancer diagnosis and had educated me about needing a medicinal dose of turmeric for it to have a beneficial effect, I decided to buy empty capsules and fill them myself. After my first go-round of dipping capsules into the turmeric bag to fill them, my fingertips looked as if I had shoved my hands into the bottom of a snack bag laced with nacho cheese dust. I made a "note to self" and used disposable exam gloves to fill them the next time. Lukas walked into the kitchen one day while I was filling my capsules, his expression obviously questioning my sanity. "What are you doing with that yellow powder?" Quick to update him on the Jains' wonderful gift and the information about turmeric and its effect on cancer cells, he brisked by me and said, "If you have another pair of gloves, I will help you!" Relieved that he knew I was not losing my mind, I assured him I was good to go, and he was off the hook from helping me with this messy, worthwhile task.

Movement was involved in the next video module, and I can still picture the doctor from the Raleigh-Durham Research Triangle in North Carolina, also of Indian descent. Although he practices Western medicine, he typically incorporates the science of movement into his treatment approach. After discussing the importance of movement in overall health, he discussed research on the body and its lymph system, mentioning trampoline bouncing to be the most effective in stimulating lymph flow and subsequently decreasing cancer risk. A vivid memory struck me—a torturous routine my mom and I sought out to get us through the Philadelphia winters with healthy bodies. Any of you who lived through the eighties or nineties will recall videos made by Jane Fonda or Suzanne Sommers wearing French-cut leotards, complemented with leggings and headbands. Personally, my mom and I were fans of Richard Simmons with his tank tops and runner's shorts. He was more relatable since my body was not quite like Jane Fonda's at age fourteen. We agreed to rise at the crack of dawn, dress in our leotards, and bounce on our own individual trampolines for thirty minutes while watching those videos. My mom would snooze on the floor during commercials, but when Richard's voice returned, we bounced with vigor as he chanted something like, "Imagine that cellulite melting away! Work that body, work that body! Feel the burn!" Now the mere thought of cellulite horrified me—can anyone relate? As a teen, body image was at the forefront of my mind, so I bounced enthusiastically, visualizing any ripples or dents in my thighs melting away.

Rewinding to the year 2013, Lukas was discovering his love for gymnastics. He frequented the indoor trampoline parks in Poway near our home, almost a daily participant. Since I considered it a healthy obsession I wanted to support, I occasionally went along to watch him flip forward and backward from tramp to tramp. After my surgical site healed and I resumed my regular activities, I would watch Lukas delight himself in movement, thinking to myself, "There are other parents out there bouncing with their children, why not me?" Since the doctor from the North Carolina area recommended it as the best cancer-preventive activity, before you knew it, I was out there doing round-offs and cartwheels, crossing my fingers that my body would remember its gymnastics skills. For my own satisfaction, and not to show off, Lukas and I would go to the gym late at night when there weren't many onlookers, and with Lukas as one of my only witnesses, I was still able to do a round-off into a back tuck or flip up until the age of fifty-two! Praying to not strain a hamstring in the process, I savored these movements, especially knowing it was stimulating my lymph flow and helping my body rid itself of toxins in the process. Who knew Suzanne Sommers and her mini-tramp had stumbled onto something pretty special back in the eighties?

The next topic was on the financial industry of cancer. Yes, in a medical professional's definition, cancer is an industry. Never had I considered this, but the host of the module mentioned it was a billion-dollar industry at that. The video stated that in only a single year they reviewed, costs for cancer care were over $180 billion—a stupefying number to me. In my opinion, there is no price tag on saving someone's life, and I believe there is a need on a case-by-case basis for surgery, chemotherapy, and radiation; but as I dove deeper into the tests and protocols, were all of them necessary? For example, breast cancer was not in my family history for anyone who was not also a smoker, but my oncologist asked if I wanted to run a genetic test and then consult with a genetic counselor. Since I adopted Lukas and I was in my late forties, I was not considering having any children from my own genetic line. In my case, I thought since I wasn't passing the gene on to anyone, and no one in my family had breast cancer, these tests and consultations weren't necessary. Aware that the BrCa gene had mutations more often found in those with Jewish ethnicity, if I were Jewish, I would have gone ahead with this incredible testing. But in my situation, I didn't feel it applied to me. So in opting out of this testing and counseling, I felt I was saving the industry some money.

This led me to study radiation and its efficacy for my type of cancer. My friend, Sharon Okamoto—with whom I discussed my cancer diagnosis—said that there was an article in *Time Magazine* about the controversial nature of stage zero cancers. In consulting this article, the benefits of radiation were questioned, so I researched medical journal articles for my type of non-aggressive, slow-growing cancer. Mind you, I had been given the choice to radiate, but could leave it as an option if the cancer were to return. In that case, it would be 100 percent recommended. The journal article I happened upon reported that for ductal carcinoma, the benefits of radiation were only 5 percent to prevent recurrence at the time of my cancer journey in 2013. While writing this book, my coworker—who had experienced the exact same type and size as my cancer and also similar in that it was hormone positive—asked her radiation specialist about its benefits after I told her about my research, and the specialist stated that radiation only decreased the return of cancer by 3 percent! This was barely any benefit at all in my opinion. The protocol was to attend daily radiation sessions for thirty days at, I am sure, a costly price. And for 3 to 5 percent peace of mind? This would not be my choice. For others, while I certainly respect their choice to use every treatment in their doctor's arsenal to battle cancer, this option did not feel necessary to me. I couldn't be guaranteed the radiation wouldn't affect my lungs and ribs in the future, and therefore, the risks outweighed the benefits. But had my radiation specialist mentioned it had only a 5 percent benefit with his detailed graphs and charts? No, he had not. When I pondered this, I also thought of the thousands of dollars I was saving the industry with my choice not to radiate.

To use my decisions about radiation and compare them to someone else's cancer situation, I am not. If I had a brain tumor and discovered that I could use a point-specific type of radiation used as treatment in the 1990s, called proton therapy—also for prostate cancer—I may have enlisted this incredible invention. I believe each individual should consider their type of cancer, aggressive or not aggressive, fast or slow-growing, consult with their oncologist, and make their best educated decision. While one of the treatments or tests could be avoided, or conversely, needed, I think educating oneself and making the best choice possible is critical.

Another module was on the incidence of cancer in the US compared to other countries. Interestingly, although the US has the most advanced healthcare, equipment, and testing available, we have the highest rates of cancer in the world. One example stated that women in the US have a greater likelihood of getting breast cancer than women in Japan. Could it be that lifestyle and surroundings have something to do with these rates? This raised many questions by the people researching cancer trends. Some researchers in the module suggested that cancer may be more "epigenetic" than genetic. Now, I had never heard the word epigenetic, and I was a biology major, so I homed in on this new word and its description. The person lecturing explained that if all your relatives lived in a big city with a noticeable pollution rate, and drank water that was contaminated, and frequently ate fried food for lunch and dinner, the majority of people in your family may get cancer. This, they said, would be "epigenetic." The gene would express itself because of the myriad stressors on its system. The true definition of epigenetics from the old-school dictionary is "the study of changes in organisms caused by modifications of gene expression rather than alteration of the genetic code itself."[6] This made a lot of sense to me. Since I was inherently susceptible to allergies and food sensitivities like my Aunt Betsy was, and since I had many stressors in my life, perhaps this combination made my genes prone to allowing cancer to invade my body. I also learned that cancer, at times, can overtake the body because of a faulty immune system that's not detecting and defending itself against defective cells, allowing them to multiply and grow. This also aligned with the fact that I was often sick as a child, more so than my sister, with repeated sinus infections and stomach flus, and even the constipation that escaped the rest of my family. My aunt suffered with sinus infections and stomach flus in a similar way. Perhaps my cancer wasn't purely genetic but developed due to a combination of continued assaults on my body and its weak immune system.

One interesting section focused on the use of essential oils in supporting the body and possibly addressing certain types of cancer. One young, vibrant girl was diagnosed with a type of skin cancer, and being old enough to decide for herself not to radiate the area, decided instead to use frankincense essential oil as her treatment of choice. Amazingly, her skin cancer retreated, and she avoided other treatment options. Interestingly, my chiropractor, Dr. Tom Stuebe, shared that he similarly used frankincense topically for an area on his head where he had been diagnosed with basal cell carcinoma, and it also disappeared. It was not proven to be the reason

_____

[6] "Epigenetics," *Oxford Languages Dictionary*.

it disappeared, but certainly, there was a possibility it had an influence on his skin cancer. I decided that if this well-known biblical oil—also given to baby Jesus as one of three gifts brought by the three wise men—possibly assisted in the vanishing of his cancer, I would try it topically on my breast. Frankincense is malodorous and strong, but I used it solely at night before I went to sleep, and Tim, wanting me to heal in any way I could, was not bothered by its pungent odor. After using it consistently for certain periods of time, the oil did not change my cancer development in one way or another, so I cannot say whether someone would benefit from it or not. Perhaps, since it has no adverse effects, one could research whether it could be of benefit for certain types of skin cancers. I haven't yet seen any research on this, but it would be interesting to know if there are any studies out there.

Another informative video was on antiperspirant use and avoiding those containing aluminum. Tim had heard something of the sort, so he was the first to initiate change in this area, ordering a particular type of deodorant that was aluminum-free. This change was more challenging for me since my job was so physical, often needing to lift patients out of bed, and working in warm rooms suited for their frail bodies. Inevitably, this led to profuse sweating as I worked. Emily Vaught, my boss in our therapy department, was also concerned about finding an aluminum-free product. Being female and aware of my cancer, she wanted to reduce her risk also. She researched deodorants, trying many unsuccessfully, and suggested a few to me, which I tried, but we both felt that most failed and left us stinky and sweaty in patient rooms. Wanting to avoid promoting a big-name brand, suffice it to say, many are now on the market advertising that they are aluminum-free. My doctors debunked this as a theory, stating it would have no influence on my risk of cancer recurrence, but I figured it couldn't hurt to avoid using aluminum products in my armpits, so close to lymph nodes, so I have chosen to use this type of deodorant to this day.

I remember at the time making a commitment to change many things, but I wasn't ready to go "all in" because, after all, the cancer was only stage zero. Julie, however, was insistent that I make more dedicated lifestyle changes and keep researching foods that would help me. To a certain degree, I did this leading up to my six-month follow-up. I followed every suggestion my oncologist had, but I figured the surgeries were behind me now, and I was making good choices. My mind wanted to believe this chapter was behind me.

I wanted to place the link to the video series here, but in trying to find it, I discovered it has been removed from YouTube. Was this because allegedly controversial statements had been made on this site? I personally felt it was educational, but try as I may, it's no longer accessible. One can only wonder why.

12

Life after Stage Zero

I made changes in my life with the goal of reducing stressors in my body. I added beneficial spices such as turmeric to my diet, decreased my consumption of sugar, and incorporated more vigorous activity to stimulate lymph flow, such as bouncing on a trampoline or going for runs as often as possible. My life now included more showers as none of the deodorants seemed to do the trick like those containing aluminum. I even tried, with intermittent consistency, the never-before-dreamed-of coffee enema, and had all the amalgam fillings removed from my teeth. I was thankful I had already gone through a root canal surgery, and felt this was behind me. At the time, my dentist said my root was intact, but the pain in my tooth and mouth was so severe, he had no other choice but to perform a root canal. I wasn't prescribed antibiotics after the procedure was complete, and I believed my mouth was clear of any additional threats. Although I did reduce my sugar intake, I didn't feel the need to eliminate it entirely, as my oncology team said it was fine in moderation. Since I no longer had stage zero cancer after the two surgeries to remove it, I didn't see it as an issue. I so wanted that to be the case.

Although Tim seemed to be much better at following all of the recommendations, and was more diligent than me with the suggested deodorant and toothpaste choices and avoidance of sugar, he continued to encourage me to follow suit. We exercised together routinely on weekends, taking walks to encourage sweating, whether it was ninety degrees or not. He would hold my hand and often help me to keep a good pace by gently "assisting" me up hills, joking that he was pulling me and I could put in a little more effort. Thankful for his support in every aspect of my healing journey, I wondered if his sacrifices would rub off on me and make it easier for me to comply with all the changes. I believed they would. But there was one weakness, deep down. Tim knew. He also knew I still wasn't ready to look at it, graciously keeping it to himself, not wanting to add to my self-imposed list of restrictions. When would it be time for this hidden area of my life to come into the light?

13

Confessions of a Chocoholic

Hidden from most of my friends and doctors lurked a seemingly innocent and benign pleasure . . . chocolate. Previously, I mentioned that I enjoyed sugar a little more than most. Now, I must share that this was more than something I enjoyed. My relationship with chocolate was an addiction. I would tell people I was a chocoholic, but inevitably, they would applaud me, laughing and joining in my club of also enjoying this dark, delicious treat too much. Part of the problem is that people brag about this, advertising it on T-shirts and mugs and making it acceptable. The problem for me began earlier in life and had seemed to be under control, but I was able to keep to myself its lurking power over me. Some friends who didn't understand my obsession even said, "I don't see that you have a problem with it, and I am around you a lot. It's not like a drinking or drug problem." Those close to me, however, were well aware of my struggle with chocolate.

When I was young, I noticed that I enjoyed the incredible taste of chocolate chip cookies fresh from the oven. Almost every weekend throughout junior high and high school, my friend Sharon Okamoto and I baked these delicious treats during our study breaks. But I always noticed I wasn't as satisfied as she. Her parents or sister were only after one cookie. I could eat a few spoonfuls of the raw dough before they went into the oven, and still desire more than one cookie. Some of you must relate—nowadays, they sell raw cookie dough in small tubs for individual consumption. I know because I have purchased them and eaten the entire tub in one sitting.

Another weakness, back in my twenties, was a particular flavor of Ben and Jerry's ice cream—Phish Food—since it contained mostly chocolate ice cream, bathed in marshmallow swirls, and chocolate fish-shaped chunks swimming throughout it. Most people can have a few bites and place it back in the freezer, but left to my own devices, or especially if I'd had a long, stressful day at work, I would resort to stopping by a store and downing the entire pint. This problem wasn't noticeable in high school because I played three sports every year, and other sports during the summer. I didn't have as much time to overeat sweets, and, if I did, I burned them off with my athletic activities. But from a young age, as early as seven, I can remember the pull toward sugared doughnuts or bakery cake icing at my friend Susie Craig's birthday parties. I believe one of my friends, Jean Oxendine, was onto my weakness, as she would ask why I wanted such a large corner piece, and may even eat her icing if she offered it to me. Also in my twenties, while working at Mercy Medical Center in Denver, my friends Rebecca Kristopeit Elrod and Nicki Kakos-Shier would notify me which floor of the hospital had a birthday cake on it. We would go together to celebrate the birthday of our colleague, and to enjoy the sweet stuff—with me always being one of the first ones in line. Little did I know the power sugar held over me and others.

Disaster was bound to strike when the stress of an internship, while earning my master's degree in physical therapy from Hahnemann University, sent me to none other than Hershey, Pennsylvania. Yes, Hershey, PA, where the streets are lined with light posts topped with alluring kisses, and the lingering scent of chocolate permeates the air. Every cell of my body cried out each day, driving home from the main trauma center, then called Hershey Hamot Hospital. Although I tried to avoid stopping at the corner store to get some Hershey's kisses or Reese's peanut butter cups, the temptation was too great. At the end of my three-month rotation, I had put on ten pounds of weight in the form of chocolate and peanut butter on my hips, legs, and torso. Since I didn't have as much time to exercise, I couldn't hide this weight gain from anyone, even myself.

When I found out I was sensitive to gluten, my sweet choices were narrowed down to mostly chocolate, and along with my problem with insomnia, I used chocolate rather than coffee to give me energy in the morning. For breakfast, I would consume it with berries and yogurt as early as 7:00 a.m., and eat it throughout the day. Aware that chocolate could, and would, interfere with my ability to fall asleep, I would attempt to cut myself off at 2:00 p.m. Even headaches would result if I ate too much. My family was so aware of my predilection toward chocolate, even my two-year-old nephew, Damiano, knew. Once, when visiting my home, my mom asked where I had disappeared to, and he said innocently, "To her chocolate closet." The mere sound of this embarrassed me and struck me right between the eyes. I needed to address this.

At church, close to this time period, we were discussing things in our lives that we felt kept us in bondage and from having a more pure relationship with God. I remember journaling that it was my battle with chocolate. Required to take thirty hours every two years on a variety of continuing education topics to maintain my license as a PT, this led me to attend a class on obesity and addiction to foods, mostly attended by nurses, to help educate their patients. My weight was fine, but I earnestly went to this class to learn why I had more of a battle saying no to sugar than most. I learned in this class that alcoholics and "food addicts" had an issue with the satiety center of their brains. Where most people could drink one or two beers, or could eat one cookie or a single cup of ice cream and be satisfied, in the brains of those with addiction problems, the area of the brain that should tell a person they should be satisfied would not "light up" appropriately, even after the addict had up to four or five cookies, or multiple hamburgers, for example. This was it! My grandfather and one of my aunts were alcoholics, and another aunt had a sugar addiction. Apparently, I also inherited that gene or tendency. This class truly helped me more than it would my patients, and from this time on, I was determined to get control of this problem. Specifically, this is the reason I had asked my oncology team if chocolate would be a problem. They had no knowledge of my intake level, and I do not fault them for saying it was fine in moderation—I hadn't told them the whole truth. A very real and potential stumbling block in my cancer recovery, I was finally ready to face it head-on. It was somewhat freeing to learn why I had a proclivity to eat more sweets than someone with a different genetic makeup, but it was not an excuse to continue a bad habit. This would be a hard lesson for me to learn.

In further research, I came across an interview by a man named Ian Jacklin with a well-known cancer survivor, Chris Wark. Ian had watched a related video and recounted what he heard. "Dr. Bernardo screamed at the camera, saying, 'If you have colon cancer, it will always, always come back . . . Why? Because you didn't address the problem . . . The problem is acidosis. You die of acidosis; you don't usually die of cancer."[7] It hit me again and hit me deeply. Chocolate is very acidic, and I ate it in small doses throughout the day. If it could contribute to digestive problems like heartburn and acid reflux, why couldn't it also set up the perfect storm in my body? Could it allow the cancer in my body to thrive, since cancer loves an acidic environment? If my choice was to heal, I not only needed to face it head-on—I needed to fight its control over me with every ounce of my being.

———————————

[7] Ian Jacklin, *I Cure Cancer: Learn How to Turn Your Body into a Cancer-Free Zone* (Independently Published, 2019), 1, 3.

14

Yes Girl

I haven't yet mentioned that, along with my tendency to eat too many sweets, I was also a "yes girl." I was a people pleaser to a fault, and for the most part, genuine about wanting everyone to be at peace with one another because it seemed harmonious this way. It also allowed me to feel less anxious. A terrible but true example of this was in third grade at Highland Elementary. My classmate, who will remain anonymous, sat next to me at our square wooden desks and was jealous, perhaps that a close friend of mine, Laurie Hess-Leasure—who was more like a sister to me—had been allowed to join me during the school day since she was visiting from out of town. This aggressive student, due to her strange jealousy of Laurie, took a pair of scissors and attempted to cut my finger, and I sat back and watched as they clamped down, getting tighter and tighter. I wouldn't have said anything until the pain was unbearable because I didn't want to upset her or lose her as a friend. Thankfully, the scissors were dull and child-friendly, and Laurie came unglued and screamed at my assaulter to stop immediately! The teacher didn't notice our commotion, currently being distracted by a group of raucous boys, but thank goodness Laurie knew how and when to say no.

This personality trait of mine carried over into my work life, at times to my detriment. Our therapy companies frequently seemed to have a short-age of PTs willing to work weekend shifts in order to evaluate new patients that had arrived on Friday or Saturday night, and I would say yes almost all the time when asked to help remedy the situation. I had one coworker, Marie Graber, who was so often willing to put in far more work than me. Since I knew she worked longer days than anyone else, I felt compelled to give her a break and see patients at her building in addition to my own. I would be out of the house before Lukas awoke and see patients at both sites, trying to make it home by lunchtime. If they were desperate, I would at times repeat this after church on Sundays. This left me without any full days off during the week. A pattern developed, and I repeated it for years, and although the days were short, I was tired, and it was still a form of stress. I learned in my research that stress was linked to breast cancer. At first, I thought to myself, *Oh, I'm not stressed*, but with nearly seven-day work weeks and full-time homeschooling at night and many days, I was only kidding myself. Not really ready to say no since the work demands continued, I kept brushing this issue under the rug, but the remnants were depositing themselves in my body. When would I learn to say, "No?" I will never know if, or how, this stress impacted my cancer journey, but if my people-pleasing nature was outranking my need for self-care, it needed to be addressed. I had only just begun.

15

That Time of Year Again

March of 2016 and my forty-ninth birthday were rolling around, and with that, my bi-annual mammogram. Thankfully, I coasted through bi-annual follow-up appointments in 2014 and 2015. Now considered at risk, I met with my oncologist and had mammograms every six months. Since I was attempting to de-stress my life, make subtle dietary changes, exercise regularly, and think positively, I truly felt this stage zero issue was behind me. Until it wasn't.

Confidently, with my favorite tech, Linda, who was still working at the same facility at Scripps, Rancho Bernardo, I assumed the positions every woman who has a mammogram undergoes. She always took great care of me, repeating the phrase, "Inhale and now hold your breath," as she captured the required images of my breasts. I always complimented her for being so thorough, and for being key in discovering the cancer cells that were so close to my ribcage they could have been missed. She completed her job positioning my arm and chest this way and that, and I was dismissed and at peace. That is, until I received another call from my oncology nurse. My OB/GYN was bypassed in this process since I was now a cancer team patient, and she uttered those words I didn't want to hear. "We detected calcifications on this breast image again, only on your right side, and we would like you to schedule a breast biopsy. After that, I will meet with you or call you with the results."

The first thing I thought was, "At least they didn't find a tumor," followed by, "Perhaps I will be like others who have calcifications but no cancer cells," and then "Why do I keep forming these calcifications?" Reminding myself that stage zero DCIS (ductal carcinoma in situ) cancer is "the best type of breast cancer to get," I promptly scheduled my biopsy— of course, on a Friday so I didn't have to miss two days of work—and mentally kept calm and hopeful. They didn't have a Friday appointment available until the end of April, but since I was determined to not take any extra days off work, the end of April it would be.

One of my friends also had breast calcifications without cancer, and another had a breast cyst that was benign; thus, I hoped for the best for myself. Entering Scripps and heading to the basement clinic, I recall getting on the elevator with other people seeking health advice of some sort, but no one was really cheery. I tried to put on a happy face to change the energy in the claustrophobic cubicle, but no one seemed to notice—everyone's heads or eyes were in a downward position.

Considering my first biopsy was nothing short of barbaric in my opinion, I was thankful the nurse said that since my calcifications were in a more central and lateral position, they would not need to go to extreme measures to get the needle in the right position. When I suggested they remove the foam pad that cushioned everyone from the metal plinth, the nurse cheerfully assured me that would not be necessary this time. Linda was not available that day, but the biopsy tech seemed more than capable, and within less than twenty minutes, I was in a satisfactory position for the radiologist to come in and insert the biopsy needle. I was pleasantly surprised, recalling that last time it had taken a two-person team over two and a half hours to get me in the right prone position for the biopsy. I was very thankful that this seemed perfunctory, and I would soon be done.

My breast was numbed prior to the biopsy in the region where the needle would penetrate. The doctor performed the procedure, removed the needle, and left the exam room. This was when I noticed faces of concern on the nurse and the tech accompanying her. They seemed to be putting quite a bit of pressure on my chest, and with my questioning look, they divulged the need for concern. The nurse said, "Kristi, the doctor did an excellent job, but as sometimes happens due to the location of your calcifications and nearby blood vessels, the doctor pierced a vessel, and you're having a considerable amount of bleeding. We will need to keep pressure on the area, and will recheck it in a few minutes." After a few minutes, the tech released the pressure on my breast, and blood squirted from my chest onto the floor. Almost retreating into people pleaser mode, and about to apologize, I stopped myself since I knew I was not at fault and simply took a deep, cleansing breath. The nurse said, "I need to wrap you tightly with an Ace bandage, and you'll need to remain here for another twenty minutes. We hope this will stop the bleeding."

Since I had worked in healthcare, in hospitals and rehab settings for twenty-five years up to this point, blood and medical challenges didn't faze me too much mentally. However, when I changed positions from supine to sitting, my body didn't follow my mind. Since I'd lost a considerable amount of blood, a shift in my blood pressure occurred, and, when I sat up, I nearly passed out. I figured the staff was probably eager to start the next scheduled biopsy, but aware of my ashen state, said I could take all the time I needed. Finally, I felt as if my head was not spinning, and the accompanying nausea faded, and I let them know I felt I could stand. Before I did, the nurse double checked for any bleeding through the Ace wrap that was restricting me to shallow, quick breaths. It was stifling! She said, "If you continue to bleed through the Ace wrap for more than a few hours, you'll need to come back to the ER later today and have that area cauterized. Wear the Ace wrap until tomorrow to fully stop the bleeding, and don't do any lifting or heavy activity for two more days."

Here I thought the FIRST biopsy was a near-disaster. Not that the doctor or anyone on the staff had done anything but an incredible job, but another anomaly had occurred during this biopsy, and I was starting to dread these tests. Prior to this, I had no idea what people had to endure for breast or other biopsies. Thankfully, I detected no additional bleeding from the site and successfully avoided a trip to the ER. Also, I was thankful I had done this on a Friday so I could return to work as planned on Monday. The nurse asked if I wanted an additional day off, but I didn't feel it was necessary. Remember, in my nature, I felt the need to say "yes" to work.

16

Anxiously Awaiting the Call

I knew from experience, if I received a phone call close to the day of the biopsy, it may not be the best news, so I braced myself for the Scripps number to appear on my phone. Results reported a week later were typically not pressing in nature, and I hoped it would come later rather than sooner. Monday, and back in the saddle at work at Casa de las Campanas rehab facility—perhaps a day too soon since I still felt a smidge of soreness in my chest area—that number appeared on my phone. In my spirit, I felt I knew the answer before the nurse uttered a word. My nurse oncologist, familiar to me from the past, said, "Kristi, I am so sorry, but we have found stage zero cancer again, and it is of the same type, DCIS (ductal carcinoma in situ). I will have our nurse care coordinator contact you to guide you and prepare you for surgery and to schedule an appointment with Dr. Torrey to discuss other options. Again, I am sorry to tell you this news, but at least it is a slow-growing cancer, and really the best kind to be diagnosed with."

That terrible feeling of dread washed over me after hanging up the phone. Thoughts flooded me before I could contain them. "Did I eat too much sugar? Has my stress level gotten the best of me and my breast? Is there anything I am doing to contribute to this, or is it just something that has overcome my body by chance?" Perhaps I will never fully know the answer to all of these questions, but I had a desire to be responsible for my actions and also do everything in my power to treat my body in the best way possible for the future.

Before I could digest the news completely, the phone calls began to overwhelm me. Although welcomed in a way, since I knew the doctors and care coordinators were doing everything in their power to prevent the cancer from spreading, there was a plethora of appointments to schedule, from a visit with my oncologist to the radiation doctor to the surgeon. Trying to keep my life as simple as possible would not be my reality for the next few weeks or months, and honestly, I did not feel I signed up for this. Making or responding to all of the necessary phone calls, I met with Dr. Melissa Torrey first. She, as always, was a refreshing delight despite the nature of my news. She mentioned that now, since we had saved radiation as an option if the cancer were to recur, she would now recommend a lumpectomy with the addition of radiation. To my dismay, I was in that minority group with a less than 15 percent return rate, I suppose. She was going to strongly recommend Tamoxifen again, being that, again, my cancer was hormone receptor-positive, meaning it was influenced by estrogen.

Taking a moment to process this information, I knew I would heed her advice to move forward with the lumpectomy. The thought of cancer cells in my body still frightened me, and I wanted them to leave my body quicker than I could say "Go!" I also knew inherently that I would not radiate, no matter what the radiation doctor said. Again, this was a personal choice, but hearing too many radiation horror stories about people's lungs and ribs being affected by radiation for breast cancer, for me, the risks outweighed the 5 percent benefit. Fear of the return didn't scare me as much as what I'd learned about the dangers of radiation, and I was hopeful that after this, it wouldn't return.

Following the protocol, I made my way to the radiation center in Torrey Pine once again, entered that stark building, and met with a radiation specialist who was different from the first but who rattled off similar statistics and facts in a cold, dry way. Not challenging his research and listening to his spiel, I let it bounce off my spirit. I left there convinced I would not take that path, despite this time being a strong recommendation.

Dr. Pamela Kurtzhals was just as effervescent as always, and although she was as disappointed as I was to be meeting for the third time, she instilled confidence that she could still maintain the integrity of my breast. She explained that the stage zero cancer was in a different but similar location, so she could not use the same incision line she had used twice before. Since the cancer was on a cellular level, she would only need to take a minute amount of tissue, and I might not even notice the change in my breast shape. Having the utmost confidence in her, I left her office and pondered the date of my upcoming surgery.

17

Summertime Sports Bliss

A wonderfully selfish but entertaining idea struck me. The 2016 Summer Olympics were about to be televised in August. I had been bored out of my mind the first few days after my first surgery, before I ventured off to Telluride, and after my second surgery, it was recommended I not exercise much. There was absolutely nothing interesting to watch on TV while I rested. I had already read Gerson's book and watched the 10-part video series my sister-in-law had recommended, so I wondered what would keep me occupied. Not wishing to watch *Wheel of Fortune* or *The Price is Right*, the Summer Olympics would be the most incredible way for me to endure my couch time, watching something I did enjoy.

Did I mention that I am a sports fan? Actually, let's add a few letters to that—fanatic! Tim always says that I am most certainly my dad's daughter. My dad was known to watch sports almost every waking hour he wasn't at work. If I entered the living room, I would say, "Hey, Dad, what are you watching now?" It could be anything from men's or women's World Cup soccer, girls' softball, the Australian Open, or any tennis tournament for that matter, basketball, football, you name it, and he watched it. At times, it could be a bit overwhelming for me and my mom—who I believe learned to tune it out over the years—but there was a part of me that aligned with sports in my innermost being. Even at age fifty-six, there's a part of me that wishes I could pick up a soccer ball and bend it into the corner like Beckham—for all you soccer fans out there who know who he is. Two weeks of Summer Olympics were just what I needed during my recovery. I just had to convince my boss, Kalynn McGhee.

Kalynn was a wonderful rehab director, and she also had my health concerns at heart. She informed me that she would prioritize my need for surgery over everyone else's summer plans. She said, "You name the date, and you go have that breast surgery."

Well, I loved my coworkers and knew that Rose Soto wanted to return to her homeland, the Philippines, that July, and that Marie Graber wanted to return to her homeland, Sweden, for Midsummer Festival (Midsommar in Swedish) at the end of June. I reasoned to Kalynn that Marie should go first to Sweden and then Rose to the Philippines, and I would be happy to wait until August for my surgery. It was not my intent to appear selfless or impress anyone by waiting. There was a method to my madness. During my two-week recuperation, I wanted to watch every minute of every day of every sport I enjoyed during the Olympics, in Rio de Janeiro, of all places. Picturing myself screaming with excitement while Bob Costas announced our men and women running across the finish line gave me joy beyond explanation!

Marie was the first to approach me, followed by Rose and Kalynn. Marie said, "Kristi, please get your surgery first, before I go to Sweden. I want you to take care of yourself as soon as you can," and the other two basically duplicated her words. But this wasn't about waiting. Watching the Olympics was the highest form of self-care I could think of! It would feed me with hope and pleasure, watching girls and guys tumble through the air, dive off platforms into churning water, or run track events, like I had dreamed of doing when I was little.

This all started for me with my dear friend Jean Oxendine, who I mentioned had shared childhood birthday parties with me, and who I had known since I was two years old. She was enmeshed in my life from church to elementary school to after-school activities. To earn a Friday night sleepover at her house, her dad, Joe Oxendine, would require Jean and me to run either the "little block" or the "big block" the following morning, three or five miles, respectively. Being that I was the guest, I was given the choice and always chose the "little block." Having his doctorate in education and being the first dean of Temple University's health, physical education, recreation, and dance departments, he certainly knew more than we did what was best for us. Due to my difficulty waking up, this morning run wasn't the early bird event to which their family was accustomed. Jean would most likely arise at 6:00 a.m., but I would wake up three hours later to find her quietly reading, perhaps making a gentle coughing noise in hopes of rousing me out of my slumber. Bewildered, if not frustrated by my inability to wake up before 9:00 a.m., they waited patiently. We would cross Susquehanna Street and run around the track at Huntingdon Junior High School, and up and down what seemed like the steepest hill in America on Huntingdon Ave! Wheezing with ruddy cheeks, I mustered my way up all the hills to keep up with the seasoned runners in this family. Dr. Oxendine would be drenched in sweat, his T-shirt soaked through and beads of perspiration pouring off his forehead and chin, but he would be beaming nonetheless that we had all obliged his wishes and run our best run to keep our bodies fit. Unbeknownst to me, he had been a Pittsburgh Pirate, and I believe he tried out for an NFL team as well. No wonder he insisted we keep active.

These weekend runs lead Jean and me to try out for the Ambler Olympic Running Club when we were in third or fourth grade. I ran shorter sprints, she ran longer distances—no surprise due to her experience with the little and big blocks—but we traveled together to practices. One runner named Kim Gallagher stood out to us, and we marveled at her ability to fly past us on the track. Obviously, she was several years our senior, in seventh grade or so when we met her, but despite the age difference, we knew her running talent was something to be admired. My dad and I followed her in the newspapers while she excelled in her track and field events at the high school level. She even won nationals and set state records in the 800 meters and the 3,200-meter relay!

Years later, after my junior year in high school, while watching the 1984 Olympics with my dad, I noticed that none other than Kim was on the track, ready to compete for a medal in the 800-meter race! Barely able to believe my eyes, my dad and I cheered her on as she finished two laps around the red track, earning a silver medal. Of note, she also won a bronze medal at the 1988 Olympics and was the only American female to medal in that distance for thirty-three years until American Athing Mu took home the gold in the Covid-delayed 2021 Summer Games. Watching someone who happened to sit next to me in the car on our way to practice a few times win an Olympic medal, and who ran on the same track as Jean and me when we were little girls with pigtails, and with white stripes at the bottom of our red shorts, was something that changed me forever. From that point on, I was nearly obsessed with watching the Olympics since I could certainly relate to the sweat and tears that went into achieving that level of success.

After a little persuasion, Kalynn, Marie, and Rose acquiesced to my idea to wait until August to have my surgery. They honestly had no idea that it was related to my desire to watch the Olympics for two weeks straight, but I knew in my heart this would help me to recover. My mind would be far away from cancer cells, and more focused on athletes from all over the globe vying for that top spot on the podium. The anticipation was so great, the idea took away almost all fear from my spirit. After calling my nurse care coordinator, Scripps had an opening for my surgery, and the date was set for August 6. Wishing the cancer to leave me and hoping for brighter things to come, I thought to myself, *Let the commencement ceremonies begin*!

18

D-Day 3.0

Tim found work in the San Diego area doing condo remodels, and finding other consistent construction jobs by word of mouth, he was able to take me to my now third lumpectomy at Scripps. As I write this, I think it is crazy sometimes that I was planning a third lumpectomy and not a mastectomy. Understandably, many people would want to just be "done with it," so to speak. My unrelenting science mind would not have it this way. I was not ready to surrender to this radical approach for cells that may remain quiet and contained forever. This is what held me back. My cancer was not yet rated a stage I, and for me, a stage zero did not pose a daunting threat necessitating such invasive measures as a mastectomy. Since my surgeon, Dr. Kutzhals, and my oncologist, Dr. Torrey, didn't bat an eyelash about me having another lumpectomy, and agreed that this was a sufficient surgery—perhaps since my second surgery was really required only because the margins hadn't been cleared during the first—I felt confident that after this surgery, cancer would be a word I could forget.

Tim and I talked about my decision, and he supported me, believing I would get through this smoothly like I had before. The cancer cells were now gathered in another area, but thankfully, they were located laterally on my breast, and this meant the incision likely would not be noticeable after the surgery. At least it wouldn't be a daily reminder of what I was going through.

Tim and I said a prayer together the night before surgery that it would go well and that this time, all the margins would be cleared, and I wouldn't need a repeat surgery several weeks after the first.

My doctor ordered a mammogram prior to surgery to ensure the marker was in the place it needed to be. This wasn't necessary during the first two surgeries, but oftentimes, a small marker is inserted during the biopsy for future imaging and surgical localization. She asked if I needed an anti-anxiety medicine prior to this, and I assured her I didn't need anything for anxiety. I felt as calm as I could be. When asked to rise from the wheelchair, I recall standing swiftly so the tech could guide my breast into the mammography clamp. I knew instantly they needed to finish quickly or I would pass out. I saw stars dancing before me and told them I was going to faint if I didn't sit down immediately. Thankfully, they got the images they needed, but with the yellowish-green tint to my skin, they allowed me to recline while they placed cold washcloths on my head. They asked if I was anxious and implied that perhaps the anti-anxiety med would have prevented this incident, but I knew it was a drop in blood pressure after standing suddenly. My blood pressure has always hovered on the low end, and this was what caused me to feel so faint. I hoped they would still be able to proceed with the surgery, since I had it so perfectly timed with my Olympic viewing schedule. To my relief, my near-fainting episode did not prevent the surgery later that morning.

Instilling confidence in me prior to being anesthetized, Dr. Kurtzhals performed her magic with precision and, true to her word, after peeling off the bandages later the next day, the incision was on the lateral aspect of my breast and not a nasty, daily reminder of the beast of cancer. I hoped this time I would fall into the category that did not have a cancer recurrence, and I continued reading not only science books, but rich novels such as *The*

Boys in the Boat, by Daniel James Brown, loaned to me by my friend Marie Croghan. Ironically, it had an Olympic-sports theme, and I devoured it in between a plethora of events.

With feelings of nostalgia, as I healed on the couch for the two weeks of doctor-prescribed sedentary activity, I was able to witness history in the making. Jamaican runner, Usain Bolt, was attempting to do what no man had ever done, and may never do again. He was going for a hat trick in the 100-meter dash, in his third consecutive Olympics, against American Justin Gatlin, who had beaten him over ten times that year in other track meets. Before the race began, Usain put his index finger to his lips to hush the roaring audience, and he made the sign of the cross over his chest and pointed to the heavens before he knelt in ready position. Justin Gatlin led at the halfway mark, and it appeared he would steal the medal from him, but Usain beckoned power from his tall, long legs and pumped his way across the finish line, earning his third gold medal in twelve years! Justin Gatlin placed second, and Andre De Grasse from Canada was a close third by an eyelash of a distance. Usain bowed to the audience, then made his signature lightning bolt pose with his arms outstretched and the Jamaican flag draped over his shoulders.

Next came the swimming events, with many, including myself, thinking that perhaps Michael Phelps had passed his prime. He was getting negative media coverage about personal struggles, and there were naysayers who doubted his ability to win. I announced to Tim that his 200-meter butterfly race was about to begin, and we both prepared ourselves for a disappointing finish. However, to our astonishment and my loud cheers that I wanted to believe willed him on, he touched the deck with his six-foot-four frame—a near sea-creature himself—with a staggering time and won gold! Tim was hooked and joined me in watching him win another four gold medals, and one silver, by just a hair, for a total of five gold medals in Rio. Combined with an otherworldly twenty-eight medals overall, this made him the most decorated Olympian in history! Words cannot express how excited I was for him to overcome his personal demons and prove everyone wrong in achieving this feat.

Another exciting athlete that I have to honor and who I fell in love with was Allyson Felix on the track. She came away with two gold medals: one in the 4 x 100 meters relay, another in the 4 x 400 meters relay, and would have won gold in the individual 400 meters had there been rules about keeping your feet on the ground. Shaunae Miller from the Bahamas would have come in second place, but at the last second dove over the finish line, seven hundredths of a second before Allyson. In my heart, Allyson was the victor, as she remained upright. To this day, I believe there should be a rule preventing runners from diving across the finish line in an attempt to place better than those with cleats on the ground. Miss Felix was a gracious loser in that event, giving all glory to God for her abilities and winning the hearts of many, including me. My summer of Olympic indulgence came to a close, but not without the pure joy of having had time to witness every event I'd wanted to see. My pleasure in reading *The Boys in the Boat* enticed me to even become a fan of the crew races, and I cheered for teams across the globe, imagining the boys from Washington State doing the same in the early 1936 Berlin Olympics.

Post surgery, this season of my life was followed by mammograms every six months, which were thankfully without suspicion, and I believed this chapter might just be behind me. Trying my best to be mindful of what I ate and periodically including a colon cleanse, I hoped that all future breast exams would be clear, and the thought of surgical interventions a distant memory.

19

Anniversary Brings Change

It had been no secret that whenever Tim's mother should pass away, he wanted to leave California and move to a slower-paced, not-so-densely-populated region. Even though his mother was still standing strong close to 88, his positive experience living near the redwood forest near Ukiah, California, beckoned him to leave his business and the bumper-to-bumper traffic of San Diego for either Colorado or Montana. I entertained the idea of Montana, being that my former Denver roommate, Beth McElroy, had moved there and loved it, but I had never really wanted to leave Colorado in the first place. Julie was living outside of Telluride, and Tim and I agreed Colorado would be a good place to start our quest for a new place to live.

Tim announced that for our ten-year anniversary, he wanted to take a trip to Colorado in the fall, and he mapped out an area to explore, including the Million Dollar Highway between Durango and Silverton. When the time came, I pictured taking a road trip with travel and sightseeing being the focus. Odd as it may sound for an anniversary trip, my mom joined us on the first leg so we could take her to Placerville, Colorado, to visit Julie and her family. The landscape that surrounded us was simply breathtaking! After a quick visit with Julie and crew and an hour or so down the road, Tim announced that he was ready to look at houses. Houses?! I thought we were taking a scenic drive! I contacted my close friend Deborah Chase, a near sister to me and a realtor in Colorado, and she connected me with Leslie Gannon-Meiring, a realtor in the Durango area. After Tim and I spent a few nights on our own in a charming bed and breakfast outside Durango, we connected with Leslie and also reconnected with my mom, who was dying to visit the properties with us. My mom and I had an established ritual of finding intriguing open house signs in San Diego and dropping in to see the architecture and design of some lovely properties. The realtors understood we had no current interest in buying, and they disguised any annoyance they might have, inviting us to remove our shoes and tour their lovely properties. We always informed them that if we had any friends looking to buy, we would spread the word for a potential sale. Now, my mom and I would no longer be "looky-loos" but potential home buyers if a particular property met Tim's and my standards.

We looked at several spectacular homes in Southwest Colorado, and one in particular caught our eye. Again, a part of me thought we were still just getting our feet wet, but after taking a tour of this home close to the Colorado-New Mexico border, complete with sweeping views of the San Juan Mountains, Tim and I were hooked. Since he was a seasoned home builder and the contractor for one of his own homes in the past, this ticked off all the boxes. It had land for a large garden and perhaps even some farm animals such as cattle or chickens. After expanding our search and Julie joining in on the hunt too, we toured a few more amazing homes in the Ridgway and Ouray areas, even finding one that had a James Bond feel with Aspens and mountain peaks at every turn.

We returned to San Diego with lots of information to share with my dad, and he decided that if both of his daughters were going to be in Colorado, he and my mom might as well join us! He proposed an idea, if Tim was ok with it, about investing in the purchase of a home with us.

After some family meetings, we found ourselves putting in an offer on the home near the New Mexico border and, before I knew it, we seemed to be transitioning from that scenic anniversary trip to an unanticipated move. On our return visit for the inspection in October of 2018, Tim and our inspector discovered a large crack where a bathroom had been added to the house and the possibility that the addition could separate from the main structure and cave into the earth. The solution from the homeowner's inspector was to squirt some orange foam epoxy into the crack to prevent this, but Tim knew the only way to solve the issue would be to pour a new foundation. Even though my heart had been set on this home, after reasonable discussions, we withdrew our offer.

A fire had been lit under my husband, and after weeks of virtual house hunting on the computer, Tim, my mom, and I again, in the dead of winter, drove to Southwest Colorado. We found about six homes we thought were worth seeing between Durango and Pagosa Springs. We found ourselves just outside of Durango, heading toward a home that would give Tim and me privacy on the upper floor, and also had a separate ground-floor unit that would suit my parents perfectly as they aged. As we drove up the snow-covered hill surrounded by pine trees, I wondered if this could be the one. Surprisingly, this home also had sweeping views of the San Juan Mountains—a feature not mentioned on the computer advertisement. It had enough room for all of us to live comfortably without another home in sight and had been sitting on the market for almost a year. There was a contract on it, but contingent on the sale of another home. Since we didn't have any contingencies, we made a competitive offer that was accepted, and I knew my days in San Diego were numbered.

Within a month of closing on the home in Colorado, Tim's mother became more ill from a diagnosis she had been given several months earlier, and she declined rapidly. Tim visited her every morning for months, helping with anything she needed, and his sister Debi had moved in to care for her one-on-one. Tim had resolved not to leave California while his mother was still battling, but she passed away in April of 2019. The door was now open for us to move.

Tim was in the middle of building a home for his sister, and contracting on other projects as well, and I felt uncertain about leaving. Little by little, my heart was tugging at me to slow down my work pace that currently compelled me to work full-time, plus some additional weekend hours. After talking with my boss, Emily Vaught, whom I adored, I found out she was going to turn in her resignation at the end of September. Fall in the mountains was a spectacular time of the year, and that was the season that seemed right for me also. Julie's son, Damiano, would be enrolling in a special school in Durango for kids with dyslexia, and if I were in the area, I could help her if she couldn't move in time for the fall semester to begin. All things considered, I informed my employer on June 1st that my last day would be September 30th, 2019. I wanted to give them ample time to find a replacement since I had worked in that building on and off for about nineteen years. What a whirlwind this year was turning out to be! My ten-year anniversary scenic drive trip had turned into a home purchase and precipitated a move. Excitement mounted in me, and I prepared myself for four seasons that were bound to include something I loved—snow. The more the better! It reminded me of those rare days in elementary school when I would wake up after a night of falling powder to see if my dad had gotten the "snow day" call from school to affirm that we could build snow forts, go sledding, and enjoy hot chocolate with marshmallows afterward. This wasn't a frequent occurrence in Philadelphia since the snow was usually more like slush or ice, but the idea of it warmed my heart. In any event, I felt ready for a change of landscape and a change in my work pace, and eagerly anticipated my return to the Rocky Mountain state.

20

That Fateful Day

March arrived, and I was keeping up with my every-six-month follow-up appointments that were part of the oncology protocol. Since it was recommended that I go one step further and have a 3D-type mammogram, mostly for cancer patients, I assumed. I called to schedule it but had to wait a little while and got an appointment in late April. Driving along the coast to Torrey Pines, I felt the ocean breeze wisping through the Juniper trees, as dew from a foggy area gently danced upon my cheeks. It was exhilarating, and with it, I felt high hopes that this test in 2019 would be clear of any dastardly cells. As anticipated, I went through the uncomfortable positions with the mammography clamp that smushed my breast like a pancake, and waited in the waiting area for the preliminary impressions from the radiologist. After a brief wait, the clinician entered the sterile room and gave me the words that were like a sweet love song to my ears. "I don't detect anything suspicious on the images we took but will send a final summary of the results." Leaving the office, the sun was already bright and high in the sky, and I felt I could inhale deeply with relief.

Later that week, I received a call from the imaging department, and they reported that no areas of concern were detected, no calcifications, and no tumors. I should continue with the next 3-D mammogram in another six months. They did note some dense tissue, but nothing to worry about. My oncologist, however, being extra cautious, recommended an ultrasound. Feeling overly confident, my first instinct was that if the 3D mammogram was negative, why would I need an ultrasound? I didn't schedule it right away and just pondered the idea.

Interestingly, while I was pondering scheduling the ultrasound, I had a coworker whose last day of work was midweek the following week, and his final treatment with a patient familiar to me was on the day after he left. Rather than cancel her appointment, I contacted the woman to ask if she minded me treating her on her last day. Thankfully, since we knew each other from previous treatments a year prior, she didn't mind. Elderly patients, in my experience, can be very particular about who treats them. Since my coworker had treated her on the eleven other sessions, and she marveled at his work, I felt very fortunate that she gave me the "green light" to finalize her care. After greeting her and reviewing her already established home exercise program, she offhandedly said to me, "Do you know I went through cancer surgery?" I responded that I was not aware of this. She went on to say, "For my age in my eighties, I really didn't have any concerns about my mammograms since they had always been negative. I had another negative mammogram, but with some dense tissue, and my doctor recommended an ultrasound. Even though I thought she was going overboard, something told me to do it, and the ultrasound found a mass. I had a biopsy, and they found cancer in my breast. I am so glad I did that ultrasound!" Chills went up and down my arms, and I felt that instant voice tell me what I needed to do next. Since I had worked with her previously for over two months, and we had formed a nice bond, I revealed that I'd just had a negative mammogram and was considering avoiding the recommended ultrasound, but her story motivated me to follow through. She was a woman of strong faith and encouraged me to follow up with the ultrasound, and we wondered if there was a bigger reason that I saw her that day. I thought to myself, *What are the chances that I'd just had a negative mammogram with orders for an ultrasound, and a woman who would not normally have even been on my schedule telling me how thankful she was for having that clarifying ultrasound that discovered cancer, after a negative mammogram*! I felt something inside whisper to me that I needed to pursue that ultrasound sooner rather than later.

Thankfully, the ultrasound was easy to schedule, and I entered the dingy, darkly lit basement of the Scripps building with an instinct preparing me for whatever was to come. As the practitioner performed my ultrasound, she kept circling her metal wand around one area again and again, and the impression I had was that the jig was up, something was about to be unearthed. The radiologist came in and said, "We've found a tumor, and I'm suspecting it's malignant. Please schedule a biopsy as soon as possible." I took a deep, cleansing breath as I processed the idea that I might have a cancerous tumor. One thing reassured me, however: I know I would have opted out of that ultrasound. Whatever was lurking would have been hidden and left to its own dark devices for another six months had I not called and rescheduled that elderly lady's appointment on a day she normally would have seen her primary therapist.

21

Medical Meltdown

Back in the bowels of the Scripps biopsy room, close to 2:30 p.m., I tried to slow my heart rate down to ready myself for my third biopsy. I had raced out of work—thankfully only several miles away—knowing I still had several patient documents to complete that evening that I hadn't had time to finish. This seemed to be my new normal, doing as much as I possibly could without taking a day off to care for myself for needed appointments. Self-care was on my radar, but I was not yet making any changes to address this driven side of myself.

My close friend Laurie Hess-Leasure called me earlier that week to talk me through this upcoming procedure and added her much-needed humor to settle my spirit. A male doctor entered the room to perform the biopsy, and as he was about to begin, I quipped, "Well, I am not sure what you will find today, but you are likely to find a chocolate chip or two," borrowing the humor Laurie had shared with me earlier. He went into controlled laughter and replied, "No one has ever joked with me the day of their breast biopsy, and that was too funny." He didn't know my friend and her ability to pull humor into a stressful situation, nor did he know the candid truth I was exposing. That part of me that felt my obsession with chocolate had something to do with what was inside my breast.

He uneventfully performed the procedure without a burst blood vessel or clamping down on my vertebral artery, as in previous years. After leaving the facility, I raced home to complete my unfinished paperwork. My mom announced she was making tacos, and I thanked her for sacrificing her time to provide a meal when I was up to my ears in work responsibilities. Remembering to ask her if the taco seasoning had MSG in it, since I had severe reactions to that, she answered that she looked at the package and it said, "No MSG." Or so we thought.

We ate dinner around 6:30, and close to 7:00, as I was finishing my last work-related document, a burning began in my fingers and hands, and then I noticed a strange sensation in my mouth. Running to look in the mirror, I noticed that my tongue appeared to be swollen and my lips were burning like my hands. I asked my mom to take me to urgent care immediately, as I could detect an allergic reaction to something. She did a double-take on the package of taco seasoning, and sure enough, there were glutamates in the ingredients, a hidden name for MSG, so companies could falsely claim there was no MSG in the package (MSG stands for monosodium glutamate). On our way to urgent care, just one mile away from where I had had the biopsy earlier that day, the female practitioner at the facility said the building was closing momentarily and reviewed my symptoms, which were worsening by the minute and said, "If it's okay with you, I'll call an ambulance to take you to Pomerado Hospital." I knew that by the time the paramedics got to me, my mom could drive me to the hospital, only two miles away, and if I was in dire straits, I would be that much closer to the hospital. Also wanting to save $1,000 or more on the ambulance ride, I told her we would drive there immediately. She was visibly frustrated that I didn't heed her advice, but we took off for the emergency room.

My mouth and tongue were beginning to swell almost to the point where my speech was garbled. I didn't realize what my appearance was like, but my mom dropped me off right at the entrance to the ER, and

I ran inside. I spoke to the man at the front desk, and I told him I was having an allergic reaction and that I felt I might vomit or faint. He took my blood pressure, which was below 70/40, and called for the med cart to get me immediately. What I didn't realize was that my entire face was covered in red welts, something my mom would tell me later. Whisked onto a gurney before having a syncopal episode and crashing to the ground, I had an oxygen meter on my finger, and a doctor came in quickly to assess my condition. Informing them that my legs and hands were now on fire, and I was finding it harder to breathe or speak, I began shaking uncontrollably. I recall saying to the doctor attending to me, "I am not exaggerating my chattering teeth or trying to look worse than I am for any reason," having been falsely accused of something of the like by another ER doctor in the past. "You are in anaphylactic shock," he said, " and I know you're not conjuring up these symptoms. We'll need to give you an epinephrine injection as soon as we can get one ordered." I repeated to him that I felt like I was literally burning from the inside out, and I looked at my arms, already hooked up to IV fluids, and noticed they were bright red from welts. My mom waited patiently by my side, sending group text messages to pray for me, and calling my boss, Emily Vaught, to let her know I wouldn't be coming to work tomorrow. Emily responded that she would have everything covered, and for me to take Thursday and Friday off as well, giving me a four-day weekend to heal before returning to work.

The ER doctor asked me kindly why the practitioner at the urgent care reported that I had left AMA, or against medical advice. "At the time," I responded, "I could sense in my body that I had little time before things went south. I know she needed to recommend that, but I felt my mom could get me to the hospital sooner than the paramedics could respond to her call, and I would be that much closer if the paramedics did need to intervene." He understood and said he would make a comment in his notes of the situation. He also asked me when my biopsy was and if I had a reaction to anything there. I reported I was fine after the biopsy, only having a reaction thirty minutes after dinner.

Wondering what was taking them so long to get the EpiPen, I thought if they waited this long to give me that injection, I certainly would have had three minutes for my mom to drive me to the emergency room. I was finally given the injection, after a forty-five-minute wait, when my breathing was beginning to get more and more labored and "tight," so to speak, feeling I had barely any airway left. Relieved for the burning and shaking to come to a halt, I tried to close my eyes and remain calm, despite the fire burning in my extremities.

This long wait triggered a memory of the ER doctor on call at this very same hospital who evaluated me over fifteen years ago when I was suddenly overcome with abdominal pain and extreme stomach distension. After crawling into my mom's room at four in the morning without the strength to stand, telling her I thought I might be having a pulmonary embolism and feeling like I could die soon, she whisked me to the ER, and the doctor accused me of being pregnant and not telling him the truth. Wondering why he would assume a person, especially one who worked in health care, would lie to him about such a matter, I insisted I was not pregnant, but he demanded I tell him what birth control I was using. Not satisfied with my answer that I did not use birth control as I was not sexually active, he sarcastically and with irritation in his demeanor asked, "Let me say it to you in simple English. Are you on the pill, a contraceptive sponge, or using a diaphragm?" I was about ready to blow a gasket but responded that I had heard him the first time, understood his question, and was sticking to my first answer that I was not using any method of birth control. After leaving the room briefly, he sheepishly returned with no apology to inform me I would need emergent surgery, and he was signing me over to the OB/GYN staff. Apparently, I was bleeding out and had lost two of five pints of blood, thus the swelling in my abdomen. This was the reason I was currently overexplaining my symptoms to the ER doctor—that triggered memory had me convinced they would think I was lying or exaggerating something. Despite my intentions to write that doctor from years-gone-by a tactful letter about how to treat patients with respect, I never did. I write this now to inspire anyone who has been ill-treated yet not confronted their medical practitioner, to be bold and write the letter so bitterness does not breed fear and other negative emotions that I now realized I had been harboring for over a decade. Thankfully, the doctor on call for this ER visit was reassuring and caring and did not make any derogatory accusations against me.

With symptoms subsiding close to 1 a.m., the doctor announced I was soon to be released. Since IV fluids had been pushed through my veins, the urge to eliminate overcame me, and I got up and walked to the restroom. Unfortunately, someone else had the same idea, and I had to stand and wait for a few minutes before the bathroom was free. Suddenly, I became lightheaded and thought if I didn't sit down soon, I would pass out and my discharge home would be delayed. Thankfully, the bathroom became free, and I grasped the IV pole to stabilize myself, making a successful trip there and back to my gurney without mentioning the dizzy spell to the doctor, so I could get back home and get some rest.

Craving sleep close to 2:00 a.m., my head lay on the pillow, but my brain spun uncontrollably, because the epinephrine that may have saved me was also a major stimulant. So much for sleep after body shock. Perhaps I nodded off for one or two hours that night, but I was thankful for the four days to recuperate.

Referred to an allergist, I had every test known to man, and the conclusion was that my severe allergic reaction was not caused by any of the meds from the biopsy, but from the glutamates in the taco seasoning. My mom revealed that she had put three heaping tablespoons in the meat, and the glutamates, disguised but truly MSG, were most likely the culprits. Also exposed was a new cat allergy, something I suspected due to sneezing when close to my furry buddies, Bandit and Mango.

A part of me also suspected that the stress of the biopsy and thoughts of cancer could have compounded the effects of the MSG. This is just a theory. But nonetheless, I felt the message was pretty clear. I needed to slow down and reduce the stress on my body and mind.

22

The Unwanted Phone Call

Since my biopsy had been midweek, I knew the phone call from my nurse practitioner in oncology was looming. It was a Monday, and I remember vividly that my friend and coworker, Tanya Becker, was sitting next to me as we worked on documenting our patient treatments. It wasn't common for us to sit together, but I realized later there was a reason. She worked in occupational therapy in our rehab department in San Diego, and we were like two peas in a pod when it came to our views on natural healing. To me, she was near guru status on this topic. Perhaps she had a photographic memory for the things she learned, as she, too, had been through battles with immunocompromised health and was always at the ready with scientific information about foods, diets, vaccines, and exercise. In this day and age, anyone mentioning the word vaccine with any hesitation is suspected of being a right-wing radical. But I beg everyone here to allow free speech, or in this case, free writing expression. Tanya was knowledgeable about vaccines due to her experience getting the measles, mumps, and rubella just after being vaccinated for this terrible triad. Doctors were perplexed, as was she, and this began her research and questioning into the effects of vaccines.

As I recall, Tanya had gotten a sporty, sexy Fiat convertible, allowing her to experience the balmy ocean air wisping through her hair and every ounce of her being. Instead, it was becoming a money pit, and due to the need for costly repairs on the inner workings of her vehicle, she had just spent part of the day at the Fiat dealership. "I had the most interesting conversation with a man named Mario today." She explained that he was sitting next to her and said, "I feel I need to share my cancer story." He went on to explain that he'd been diagnosed with metastatic cancer that had begun in his prostate and migrated to his liver. He was so excited because he decided to go on a strict diet along with other treatments, and his cancer was no longer present. He wanted to share with others what he did.

No sooner did she finish explaining this to me than I got that phone call. Instinctively, I knew before I looked at the number that it would be my nurse practitioner with my results. Sure enough, there was the Scripps number, and when I answered, she said, "Kristi, I am sorry to report this, but this time your cancer has advanced from stage zero and you have invasive ductal carcinoma, stage I, about one centimeter in size. I will have the triage scheduler call you to set up appointments with the surgeon and the radiologist." I thanked her for her phone call and told Tanya immediately. After exchanging a hug, she said, "Maybe there was a reason I was at the Fiat dealership, sitting next to a man whose cancer was cured. I have his number; you should call him as soon as you can." The reason I was sitting next to Tanya became obvious, and I didn't hesitate in calling Mario later that day—we set up a meeting for the following week.

Walking into Panera to meet Mario, I noticed a man carrying a plastic container holding lots of vitamins. I guessed this must be Mario, and we found a table and sat down. He was so motivated to share his story with me! He mentioned that when he was in the hospital, a doctor whose father was failing in his cancer battle had been invited to come and seek his advice for the sole purpose of asking Mario what he was doing to amazingly reverse his cancer. Mario said, "I hope to share my journey with anyone who will listen! Kristi, if you choose this method, you have to commit.

After talking to a medical clinic in Mexico, I went on an alkaline diet. I only allowed myself a handful of berries in the morning, and I took lots of vitamin D and C, hydrogen peroxide in specific doses, and also a solution made in Mexico that is supposed to slow down or reverse cancer growth." I noticed that his plastic container was well-used and tarnished with brown droplets, perhaps the solution he described he bought in Mexico. He said, "My cancer was advanced, and if your tumor is just in one place and one cm, I believe you can heal too."

Thanking him for his time and information and his incredible story, I told him I would call him with updates after some of my doctor's appointments. He said he would pray for me and, after I wrote down all of his suggestions, we parted ways. While driving home, I considered the timeliness of meeting him and getting this valuable information just days after my new diagnosis of stage I, invasive cancer. It was no longer stage zero, so I needed to address it from a more serious perspective than "this could become a tumor." I would do everything in my power to overcome it.

23

Placed in a Box

Scripps had the best coordination efforts in helping me to schedule appointments, and again, I was making that familiar drive to Torrey Pines to meet with the radiologist first, and the surgeon directly after that. Since I was not entertaining the idea of radiation, that appointment was not remarkable or memorable, other than a female doctor in a white lab coat telling me those familiar recommendations for thirty days of radiation following a lumpectomy. Since I had researched this and found that radiation only benefited me by 5 percent at the time, I was not planning on going down that path. Thus, I was disengaged and attending the appointment as a formality to please the oncologist so she didn't think I was deviating from the path of recommendations. Now it was time to meet with the surgeon. My previous surgeon, Dr. Kurtzhals, had moved away, so I was assigned to another breast specialist. Upon meeting her, I sensed a cold, businesslike demeanor. After reviewing my surgical history, now including three lumpectomies, I had a feeling she would be driven in a radical direction, and I was right. In her defense, why wouldn't she want to make a radical approach to provide optimal outcomes for me?

She started to discuss her strategy and said, "Since you have had stage zero with several lumpectomies in the past, I do believe it would be best if you had a mastectomy. I will consider a partial mastectomy, but it will also disfigure you." I knew that if this had been my first rodeo, a lumpectomy would be recommended for a stage I tumor, but since I had been down this path before, I was prepared for this to have been her suggestion. Being that my research at the time indicated radiation only benefiting me by 5 percent, I mentioned that I was hesitant about radiation. Not mentioning this statistic to her, she commented, "If you choose not to radiate, I will not do your surgery." Wow, this response caught me off guard! Where was the patient's choice in this process? In her opinion, I had no choice. Next, she repeated, "Since you have had multiple lumpectomies, I would recommend a mastectomy." Realizing that this did make clinical sense, I commented, "Let me think about this for a moment," to which she responded, "Oh, you are one of those. You are not ready to let go of your breast." *One of THOSE? She's so devoid of sensitivity*, I thought to myself. Letting my breast go was not just a cosmetic act. Little did she know I had written the post-mastectomy protocol for the therapy department at my first PT assignment. Surgeons wrote orders for PT to evaluate post-mastectomy patients and treat them in the initial stages after breast and lymph node removal. The pain could be debilitating, and not just for days. Since the muscles in the "pecs" were involved, some women had pain radiating into their ribcage, shoulder blade, and back, and some had residual lymph-edema, needing lifetime management with a compressive arm sleeve. This was not just a split-second decision for me. So to be called "one of those" was repulsive to me. Feeling pressured, I scheduled the mastectomy for the end of August, but as I drove home, a flood of tears erupted from me. In my soul, I knew I did not want her to touch my body. Not with an approach that did not give me the freedom to opt out of radiation or select a partial versus a full mastectomy.

When I arrived home, I was thankful Tim was already there. He gave me a warm embrace and asked, "How did the appointment go? I can already tell it wasn't the best." After I told him what she said, he responded,

"She will not be your surgeon. I do not want her to touch you, not with that attitude. If we have to drive somewhere else to find your previous surgeon, we will, but I don't want someone like that to treat you."

Feeling like I had been placed in a box of misfit toys, I was at least assured that Tim understood and supported me, and I could find a different surgeon if this was what I needed. After talking before we went to sleep, I knew I would not see her again, and this gave me a sense of peace. I prayed and asked God to guide me in this process.

The next morning, I woke to a distinct voice in my spirit that said, "Do not do this surgery right now." It was clear and definitive. It was the answer I needed. I had called my friend, Chrissy Stone, and we planned on going for a walk that morning. As I walked up the hill past the chaparral on my way to her house, the dense morning coastal fog dissipated, and the sun began to pierce through. A wave of peace washed over me, and I sensed I was on the right path. As soon as I saw Chrissy, I gave her a big hug, which she happily returned. I told her what the doctor said and how I heard a voice from within and probably from above, guiding me not to have surgery with this surgeon. She listened patiently and said she also wouldn't want someone with that personality working on her. She added she wasn't sure she would be strong enough to walk away from the surgery right at this time, but she supported me in my decision and would be there to pray for me and with me. Later, she mentioned that she shared this with her husband, and he agreed he would support her if she ever had to face this scenario.

As I returned to my house, the peace remained with me, and I knew I had a long road ahead, but I also knew it would not include a female physician who called me "one of those."

24

Confirmation x Three

My friend, Kristen Moriarty, a former coworker and an occupational therapist whom I had worked with at The Remington rehabilitation department, called me and asked if we could meet for lunch. I gladly agreed, and we arranged to meet in the Rancho Bernardo area as soon as possible. We met at a restaurant and enjoyed a light meal, and, after I told her about my cancer challenges, she said, "Kristi, I just met a woman who said she was open to talking to you. She has an amazing cancer healing story! She's an area realtor who showed me a home recently and talked to me about everything related to her breast cancer. If you want to talk to her, I have her number, and I told her you might call." Eager to speak with this woman, I accepted her number. Kristen said she would support me in this journey and told me to let her know how the conversation went if I got in touch with her.

Not hesitating, I reached out to this woman named Christine and came to find out she was now living in Costa Rica. She and her husband, Theo Hanson, scheduled a call with me, and she told me her story. She had been overwhelmed with work in the San Diego area and mentioned that her husband was not eating the right way and had health issues also. Just before leaving on a trip they had planned, she found out she had ductal carcinoma, just as I did. When I asked her the size, she said it was 1.5 centimeters, and mine was 1 centimeter, so they were similar in size. Next, she mentioned that it was HER2 negative, and I thought to myself, *So is mine.* She continued that her cancer was slow-growing (same as mine) and that she was still planning on doing a mastectomy, but, explaining to the surgeon that she and Theo had a sailing trip planned in a few weeks, she asked, "Do you think we could go on our sailing trip and enjoy that before the surgery or would that be too risky?" The surgeon confidently responded, " I have been researching your cancer for over ten years, and because it is a non-aggressive, slow-growing form of cancer, you could easily delay this procedure. I believe you have one to three years before it would be of danger to you, so yes, go on that trip and plan your mastectomy when you return." Relieved, she and Theo set out on that three-month sailing trip and went to an area near Costa Rica. While there, they met another sailor who had had amazing health results from a diet change, and felt this was more than a serendipitous meeting, so they both radically changed to a vegetarian diet, including juicing. They were away from the daily stressors of their rigorous jobs and focused on healing. Upon their return to do medical testing, Christine did a repeat MRI to find that her cancerous tumor was gone! Theo added that his heart condition improved, his cholesterol went down, and he'd lost upwards of forty pounds. They had started a healing center in Costa Rica and invited me to come. Amazed by her story, and that we had the same type, size, and estrogen-fed cancer, I felt that if she could heal, why couldn't I? They gave me the name of "Chris Beat Cancer" and said they had met him and he had a wonderful healing story and video series, and that I should look into it.

On another occasion, after telling one of the nurse assistants at the rehab center where I worked that I had breast cancer, she said, "Oh, I wish you could talk to one of my friends named Maria, who had an advanced breast cancer with tumors in both breasts. She wanted to try to heal naturally, and perhaps I could connect you both. The only thing is, she only speaks Spanish." This was not a problem since I lived in San Diego, where many people speak both Spanish and English, so we arranged a phone conversation during one of my breaks, and I had someone interpret for her. She explained that she didn't want to have a bilateral mastectomy, but since it was already in both breasts, the doctors didn't offer any other alternatives. She said she prayed and felt guided to drastically change her diet. She eliminated all sugar and ate mostly raw vegetables and a little bit of meat. After further testing a few months later, she found her tumors had shrunk, so she continued her diet and was cancer-free a few months after that. I got off the phone and felt so encouraged! To talk to someone who had been healed of cancer in both breasts, with tumors that were more than one cm at that, placed confidence in me to give this natural approach a shot.

I hadn't yet called my surgeon to cancel the appointment, and I had many nervous friends and relatives who I could sense were urging me to take action and have the surgery. Of course, they wanted the best for me and didn't want me to linger and waste precious time, given the diagnosis. This was my hope as well, and my mind was swirling with anxious thoughts while trying to do my best at work as I battled with this decision.

The next interaction that transpired still intrigues me to this day. There was a relatively young female patient on my schedule who had suffered a stroke with barely any noticeable physical deficits, except for severe expressive aphasia, meaning she could not articulate what she wanted to say. I treated her that entire week, challenging her with functional exercises, but her expressive aphasia didn't improve. Since navigation of a facility and "path finding" were something therapists address in rehab, I decided to walk with her in our building and see if she could find her way back to her room. As we walked, she desperately insisted with her garbled communication that she wanted something the nurses weren't giving her. I thought if I took her to our facility's "convenience store," perhaps she would find it there. She scanned the shelves hunting for what she needed, and kept trying to say what she needed, to no avail. Not finding what she desired, she was exasperated. I unsuccessfully asked questions such as, "Is it deodorant, shampoo, or over-the-counter medicine that you need?" Making our way down the flight of stairs and back to her room, I noticed the safe and steady alternate step pattern she was taking, and that she was able to successfully find her way back to her room, making turns and passing through doorways without any prompting. It was a busy day, and I hadn't slept well, and my eyes were dry and irritated, as if tiny crystals of sand were rubbing against my eyelids, and I said, "Let me stop in our department and get some eye drops." Well, she about had a heart attack, frantically stammering with her hands, pointing to her eyes and indicating that was it, she wanted eye drops! I asked her if that was what she'd been trying to say, and she nodded excitedly that I finally understood what she wanted. So relieved, we walked to the nurse's station to explain what she had been trying to tell us all day, and headed back to her room. I needed to run to another doctor's appointment, and so I mentioned this, and she grabbed onto my arm and clearly said, "Anxious," and pointed to me, then expressed the words that left me speechless, "Natural healing." I was completely flabbergasted. She spoke, and she spoke clearly, and directed this to me, without knowing anything other than that I was trying to run to a doctor's appointment. She didn't know it was for cancer, and she didn't know I was debating about this mastectomy and a natural approach to healing. A calm washed over me that I cannot explain, and I knew I had my answer.

What were the chances that soon after receiving my diagnosis, I would meet and talk to three different people, Mario, Christine, and Maria, within weeks, and hear inspiring stories of recovery? Then, to have this verbally compromised patient who hadn't uttered an understandable word all week, express with clarity about natural healing intended for me, I felt God guiding me to walk on this path. I talked to Tim and my family, and my dad offered to pay for me to go to Costa Rica to experience Christine and Theo's program and dietary suggestions. Lukas and Julie also encouraged me to go, but honestly, I didn't want to burden my dad with this. I had another idea in mind. Tim was planning to go and work on the house we had purchased in the Durango, Colorado area, and I thought to myself, *Why don't I see if I can join him*? I knew it would mean I would need to cancel my upcoming mastectomy, but after meeting or speaking with all of these people that had crossed my path at just the right time, I knew this was a step I was ready to take. My boss, Emily, agreed to give me the time away from work, and I planned a quick, five-day trip to Durango to give me time to digest some of this new information.

I made the dreaded phone call without having to talk to the surgeon and explained that I would be moving soon and wanted to pursue care in that area. Without any resistance from the surgery scheduler, I was free from thoughts of that insensitive surgeon operating on me.

25

❖

Getaway

The thirteen-plus-hour drive to Southwest Colorado with Tim was restful and rejuvenating. Absorbing the changing landscape from sea level, through the desert, and then land owned by various Native American Indian tribes near the canyonlands was fascinating. I had traversed this path before, but this felt different. Realizing I would be leaving the San Diego area and the ocean climate for the majesty of the mountains was bittersweet, and it would be happening in only another month. But with it came an excitement, a resounding peace. As we passed the painted and layered rocks that talked to me about the winds and waters that had swept over them near Tuba City, Kayenta, and Teec Nos Pos, Arizona, a confidence filled me that I would heal in some way.

Tim worked every day on our future home, while I had time to go on walks and meander into our new, little town of Bayfield, and farther out, Durango, to find things like my new grocery store or the cheapest gas station, and a new favorite restaurant. This was a challenge since I was moving from a city with almost one and a half million people to a town with only 2,800 people. Actually, it wasn't that hard to find a favorite restaurant there since there were only six to choose from at the time.

One day, while I was on a hillside that overlooked the La Plata mountain range, I felt the courage to make the phone call that Tim and I had discussed on our drive. Although I had already called the surgeon to cancel the mastectomy earlier that week, I needed to call the Scripps Oncology department to tell my doctor, whom I really admired, that I would not be following up with her or her team any longer, but moving soon and pursuing medical treatment in Colorado. This phone call was less painful than I had imagined, as the move gave me an out. I wouldn't have to tell them I was not pursuing the surgery or radiation as they recommended. Since I avoided confrontation at any cost, I'm not sure how I would have handled it had I been going "rogue" while remaining in San Diego, but I didn't have to worry about it since this move was organically happening at the same time as my newfound diagnosis. As I looked out over the 14,000-foot mountains, with the phone call behind me, an assurance that I was taking the right path erased the anxiety of the past few weeks and the myriad appointments I had attended.

While sitting at a local Mexican restaurant eating a hearty salad with overly grilled and somewhat charred chicken, Tim asked me if I felt relieved the surgery was canceled, and if I was enjoying time away instead. Responding that I never felt more sure of an answer than now, he held my hand, a warm expression gracing his face as he munched on chips and salsa, comparing them to those he liked just over the Mexican border from San Diego, where he'd lived most of his life. We talked about the slower pace of life as we made our way home, past cows and goats and fields of hay that our new neighbor had in rows on her land. Yes, we weren't in Kansas anymore, as Dorothy from *The Wizard of Oz* had said, but I think we were going to like it here.

26

Alternative Strategies Intersect

J ust prior to our trip to Colorado, my friend Erica Viviani and her husband Jerome Stewart—who both had an interest in seeking the "root cause" for illnesses—called to tell me they had watched a video of a naturopathic doctor interviewing a woman who had healed from cancer naturally. They wanted to know if I was open to watching and listening to it. Of course, I welcomed it and didn't hesitate to listen to it that same day. Interestingly, I recognized the woman as being someone I, too, had come across in my research. Her name was Nasha Winters, and she had been diagnosed with stage IV ovarian cancer when she was in college. Being that her choices for healing were slim to none, she opted to try a different approach since she had nothing to lose. She ate rice and lettuce—which she now knows would not be the best diet—but amazingly, she healed from her cancer!

I was truly in awe of her amazing story, so, of course, I was excited to watch the video they sent. Nasha was being interviewed by Dr. Stengler, and it was clear that they approached cancer and healing from multiple perspectives. Not delving into the specifics of the video, what struck me was Dr. Stengler's Minnesotan accent. I had a thing for accents and liked to pick up on the sounds and see if I could guess where people were from.

Having grown up in the Philadelphia area, I was a pro at detecting an East Coast or Philly/New Jersey accent in a heartbeat. Disappointed with the idea that he lived in Minnesota, and seeing him for a consultation was likely out of the question, I decided to look him up anyway and was stunned to find he was located in Encinitas, California, just half an hour away! This, to me, was not a mere coincidence, but guidance toward my healing path, and I scheduled an appointment with his partner, Dr. Mark LaBeau, since Stengler was booked for months. Securing that appointment just before I went on my trip to Colorado gave me new hope in my ability to heal without a radical surgery. During my meeting with Dr. LaBeau, I learned that their approach was to combine Western and Holistic practices and to never go against the recommendations of any oncologist. After blood tests to look for deficiencies were complete, he recommended I start the Mediterranean diet, take various supplements, and pursue vitamin C IVs (IVCs)—yes, high doses of vitamin C given intravenously. Never having heard of this latter treatment strategy before, I decided to investigate before jumping in. I googled some related documentaries and found that it could be used as an adjunct to any other cancer treatment. Debunked by many doctors in Western medicine, it was considered controversial. Only learning why later in my reading, I decided it couldn't hurt and was tested to see if it was safe for me. After getting the green light, my boss Emily and I carved out time in my schedule for me to leave work for the two to three-hour vitamin C infusions. One day, while getting the infusion, I sat next to a woman who was battling stage IV breast cancer, and although also receiving chemotherapy, her oncologist had approved her to try this in concert with those treatments. This was encouraging to see both doctors working together rather than opposed to each other. Later, I read in one of Dr. Stengler's books that Linus Pauling, who won two Nobel Prizes, conducted research in the 1970s with Dr. Ewan Cameron, using IVC at a dose of ten grams daily for ten days, followed by daily doses of oral vitamin C. Used in terminal cancer patients, it had a four-fold increase in life expectancy.[8] Unfortunately, Dr. Stengler explained that while researchers from the Mayo Clinic did perform studies on advanced-stage cancer patients, they only used oral vitamin C at ten grams. Their conclusion was that this vitamin C treatment had no statistical benefit, but they clearly had not conducted the comparison studies in exactly the same way. The medical world, however, welcomed this study as the gold standard that vitamin C treatments were of no benefit and have been dismissed to this day by conventional medicine.[9] Since most of us learned in middle school about Linus Pauling and his research related to the benefits of high doses of vitamin C, information like this frustrated me, yet the medical community has not been willing to open their minds to these complementary types of interventions. It was encouraging that the young woman next to me had a doctor who was open to this treatment—perhaps because she was in such a late stage—and my ongoing hope is that more doctors will consider looking at myriad approaches to best treat their patients.

I scheduled a few more of these sessions right up until a few days before moving to Colorado, and one day, when receiving the IVC treatment, I recognized Dr. Stengler from the video I had seen. He approached me and his other patients and asked how I was doing. I replied that I was doing well and also that I would be moving to Colorado shortly. I went out on a limb and asked if he knew of any naturopathic doctors near Durango, thinking I would likely need to travel to Denver to receive the continued IVC treatments. I was shocked when he said there was a clinic in Durango called Namaste that had been started by Nasha Winters. "What?!" The woman I had listened to and admired for her natural healing of stage IV cancer started the clinic that he recommended, and I could easily access it

[8] Richard Stengler, NMD, *The Stengler Cancer-Reversing Protocol: Your Personal Guide to the Most Powerful Natural Cancer Therapies* (Baltimore: Health Revelations, 2014), 3.

[9] Stengler, *The Stengler Cancer-Reversing Protocol*, 3–4.

without driving six hours! This was just one more incredible confirmation that I was on the right path. For me, too many things were lining up to not be mistaken as divine direction. I would find the Namaste clinic she established and continue on my path to natural healing.

27

Return to the Rockies

There was a part of me that never wanted to leave Colorado after I adopted Lukas. I wanted to live in this rugged, majestic state forever, and wanted to raise him there. This was not to be, but after raising Lukas in San Diego and meeting Tim, a native of San Diego, I was now getting to return to the state I had never wanted to say goodbye to. I felt assured and understood by something beyond me that knew this place filled my soul. Tim was the one who had initiated the move I didn't even know I secretly yearned for, further confirming that this was the right step at the right time.

There were days in the months to come, however, when I passed rows of hay tightly rolled or in stacks, and fields of cows or goats, when I hadn't met any friends and was truly alone. "What am I doing here, God?" Wasn't I a city girl who knew nothing about the lifestyle of a rancher or cattle community? On October 1, with my car packed to the brim with luggage and boxes of necessities, I left San Diego with my mom. Erica and Jerome followed a few days later, to help me adjust and settle in, their car filled with belongings that didn't quite fit in my vehicle. Tim was busy finishing the rebuild of his sister's home from practically the bottom up, which had been drastically delayed by about a year due to San Diego's city restrictions. He wouldn't join me until spring.

Along with Julie and Damiano, we stayed just outside of Durango in a cabin in Lightner Creek, with Aspen trees changing in their splendor, and pine trees standing tall. Julie would be living here and also near Telluride until she could permanently move to the area. Damiano was starting sixth grade at a small school for dyslexic children in Durango, while Tatiana finished her tenth-grade school year in Telluride. I gladly watched over Damiano, getting him to school while Julie was in Telluride with Tatiana. Any extra time spent with my nephew was welcomed, and I often referred to him as "Love Child" and "Easy Like Sunday Morning." No drama, no attitude, no fuss, just love exuded from him, so unless he was at school or back in Telluride, I wasn't completely alone all of the time.

Before my mom, Erica, and Jerome and their precious dog Peaches headed back to San Diego, we all took a drive through the valley of Durango, following the path of the historic train that many travel to experience. We ascended the mountains near the Purgatory ski slopes on the "Million Dollar Highway," named perhaps due to the cost of the road, but there were also million-dollar views of Colorado blue skies and sunshine-drenched mountain peaks—truly priceless. We made it to Silverton at 10,000-plus feet, and thankfully, none of us were struck with the dreaded altitude headache. We soaked in the beauty of the changing colors that many traveled to witness. Saying goodbye to Erica, whom I'd met in Denver and spent eight-plus years there enjoying our single twenties life, and then living in San Diego for almost twenty years with her, was sad for me, but I knew we would remain close, as we had experienced so much of our lives together. So thankful she and Jerome were able to help me adjust to my new home, I wished them farewell with an open-door invitation to return. They encouraged me to continue my pursuit of natural treatments, having introduced me to Dr. Stengler, and assured me they would visit.

The next day, after taking Damiano to his new campus for dyslexic children, the Liberty School, I learned the staff could use help listening to kids while they read. Always one who enjoyed supporting youth, I volunteered as often as I could, and met some wonderful kids who struggled to read but were making great improvements as far as I could tell. Damiano was thoroughly enjoying the school for dyslexia, never complaining once about going. He'd actually become physically ill from the anxiety of attending public school, as he was chastised for not being able to spell simple words, and would be sick to his stomach for days on end. At the school in Telluride, the teachers were not yet trained in how to address his disabilities with reading and writing. The Liberty School, however, brought nothing of the sort upon him. He loved seeing his new friends and learning from his teachers in a style that encouraged his way of learning. He met one boy from Bayfield named Rance, who, thankfully, he could carpool with on occasion, and who roped cattle or bulls competitively. After Damiano witnessed this firsthand, he felt roping and riding bulls was a little too risky for him, and he would stick with soccer.

While Damiano was in school, I contacted Namaste and got an appointment sooner than I expected. Since Dr. Stengler's office had done some initial testing, they could schedule me to continue the vitamin C IV treatments right away, and then schedule an appointment with Dr. Stacey Mulkey at her first available slot. I was greeted by a vibrant woman named Cyd, who coordinated my care there and instructed me to continue the protocol I had begun in San Diego, including the remaining IV treatments, the number of which would be decided upon by Dr. Stacey after I met with her. Once there, a nurse named Aaron administered my IVs and encouraged me with his godly spirit to seek natural healing if possible. Since I hadn't yet found work, I had time to attend these two and a half hour IV infusion sessions without feeling rushed.

I met with Dr. Stacey for my appointment, and we did hormonal testing and blood work, which identified that it would be helpful to begin a supplement that would help me maintain hormonal balance and breast health since my cancer was estrogen-fed. She also recommended I take something called Turkey Tail mushroom supplements. Since there were so many supplements, I took the Turkey Tail at her suggestion for a time, and then, not realizing its value, thought I could do without it and save a penny or two. She was warm and understanding, and also inquired about my stress levels and work history. Since there was evidence suggesting a link between stress and breast cancer, she wanted to make sure I had a work-life balance conducive to healing. She recommended I follow the diet Drs. LeBeau and Stengler suggested—a Mediterranean diet without sugar—and to have a follow-up breast MRI in the late winter.

I felt assured under her care, as cancer treatment was her focus and what she researched continually. She mentioned that Nasha Winters, who started the practice, was now speaking internationally about cancer healing, and left the clinic in their hands. I gathered all of the supplements she recommended and followed all of her advice strictly. Cyd and Dr. Stacey mentioned that in their experience, the MRIs in Durango could be quite costly, and by going to Denver, I might save quite a bit of money. Since I was not yet working, I had no medical insurance. Yes, I was that someone who had worked in healthcare for over twenty-five years and had no medical insurance. The cost of COBRA coverage was astronomical, and so I was paying for everything out-of-pocket, hoping I wouldn't get into a car accident or have some other medical catastrophe. This was a sad state of affairs as far as I was concerned, that others who had never worked were covered better than I was, but I would try to find reasonable coverage once I began to work again. After I delved into the cost of MRIs, I found that the out-of-pocket cost for an MRI in Durango was close to $2,000. If I traveled to Denver, it would be just under $500—a savings close to $1,500! I was thankful for their advice and would pursue a follow-up in Denver.

One day, while waiting in my car for Damiano to finish soccer practice on a cold and blustery fall day, I reached out to my friend Monica Pelle, RD, CPT, whom I'd met in San Diego. I told her about my cancer recurrence, and she, being a "health coach," asked if I had heard of the use of essential oils for cancer. Mentioning to her that I had heard about and used frankincense already, she encouraged me to use several oils to combat the cancer and boost my immune system. Knowing that the application of multiple oils would be rather pungent, I figured it was the perfect time to experiment with them since I was alone for most of the day with Damiano in school, and Tim was still in San Diego. Monica shared an arsenal of information and gave me several protocols, one for cancer, one for a possible flu, and one for allergies. She recommended that I use frankincense, rosemary, lemongrass, copaiba, geranium, lavender and peppermint, some on my feet, some on my spine and elsewhere, and to apply them all at once. This was a ritual I employed right before I would go outside to walk in the hills near my home, removed from people and anyone I might offend by my aromatic potpourri. Interestingly, I noticed that I felt energized by these oils, so no matter what their effects were, I felt I had benefited from them during this solo season in Durango.

Due to the strong aroma from these oils, I applied them in a separate bathroom from the one I commonly used and had placed a greeting card in there that I enjoyed looking at, given to me by my friend and coworker, Gina Derham. She gave it to me on my last day at Casa de las Campanas, and it had a picture of a gopher with his arms outstretched to the mountains and the heavens, with words above its head exclaiming, "Be Healed," in big, red letters. Inside it said, "Can I get an Amen!"? This card meant more to me than Gina's mere gesture of care and concern, for the words she wrote filled me with hope, fueled me with inspiration, and could fuel someone else's journey as well. She penned, "When we thank God for things we've prayed for, it's called gratitude. But when we pray for and thank God for things we need but haven't already received, it's called faith. You are already perfect, whole, and healed." Each time I read this card that I have kept to this day, along with others with words of encouragement and prayers for healing from my soul sister, Michelle Rosenblum and dear friend Linda Davis, I was reminded that I needed to press toward the belief that healing was on its way, even though I couldn't quite see it yet.

28

Serendipitous Sunday

One day in October, after picking up Damiano from school, he asked if we could find a pizza place for dinner. Not knowing what Bayfield had to offer that would satisfy his mature palate for pizza—his dad Nicola being a chef from Italy—we headed into town on a quest for Italian food. Surprisingly, I spied a food truck advertising "Eepa's Pizza" only ten minutes away. With only six restaurants in the entire town, we were delighted to find this traveling treasure, especially since they said it was handmade in a wood-fired oven. Since Damiano knew I wasn't eating any gluten on my "cancer diet," he asked me if I would be able to find anything, and I assured him I could, after spotting a salad on the menu. A lovely teenager welcomed us by looking at Damiano and saying, "Hi, handsome! What can I get for you?" He ordered a Supreme Wolverine, and I got the salad, and as we waited for our food, I noticed she was wearing a shirt that said, "Life Church." With no other customers in line, I asked her where the church was. "Oh, if you came from that direction on Bayfield Parkway, you passed it up on the hill on the right." I commented that I'd seen it, and she said, "We have a youth group too, and if you (looking at Damiano) want to join us, we have really nice people in it. You both should come sometime." I told her that I would see her there soon and thanked her for the invite. Her name was Raissa, and I was truly touched by her exuberant and welcoming spirit. Back at the house, Damiano finished the entire made-for-one pizza and commented that he was surprised that in such a small ranch town like Bayfield, he could find pizza almost as good as his father's.

The following Sunday, taking Raissa's suggestion, I made my way to the Sunday service at Life Church. The quaint church was the polar opposite in many ways to Green Valley Church I'd attended in San Diego. Green Valley was in an industrial park in a large concrete block-like building with no natural light or windows, perhaps 500 members, two services, and large screens to project song lyrics and sermon notes. Life Church was situated on a hillside with horses grazing in the distance, an apple tree that had already yielded its fruit, and windows on three sides of the building. The congregation was small, perhaps forty people, with one service and two small projection screens. Thankfully, their core beliefs were similar, and the worship music, led by the senior and assistant pastors, was contemporary, which I liked.

The senior pastor—noticing I was new to his church—introduced himself to me and was warm and inviting. After finding a seat, I couldn't help but notice that the church had sweeping views of the mountains behind and to the east of the pulpit, and I could watch birds soaring and gaze upon the mere beauty of the land. After brief announcements about youth group meetings and activities, and following a few songs, some familiar to me and some not, the pastor, Chris Bernard, was about to preach when something caused him to hesitate. He said, "This feels a bit bold, and I wasn't going to say anything, but now I know I have to. This morning, God spoke to my heart about this church and told me someone here has cancer, and that they are going to heal, and we are going to have a cancer-free church. Does anyone here today have cancer?"

Overwhelmed by his words, I glanced to my right and left and behind me, and no one else was coming forward to say they had cancer. Here I was, a first-time visitor to the church, and I felt it was odd that even with a small congregation, I would be the only one that day who would have cancer, and that God had given Chris that message. I raised my hand and, with tears streaming down my cheeks, revealed that I had cancer. He asked me if the church could pray for me, and without hype or dramatic display, he simply prayed for the power of God to heal my cancer and for this church to be cancer-free.

I felt the power of that prayer flow through my body, and it gave me hope and faith that I could heal naturally, without the mastectomy. I understood that others required this surgery as they had more aggressive and later-stage cancers, but I felt in my soul that was not to be my journey. I left Life Church that day knowing I would return and that I had found a church that felt like home in that first visit.

For those of you who don't attend church, when people like me who do enjoy going to church look for one after a move, we call it "church shopping." In San Diego, Lukas and I visited five or more churches over several months before we settled on Green Valley Church, mostly guided by my son's fear of highways. Since he was from an orphanage in a small farming village and had only been in a car a handful of times on two-lane roads, if anything, he dreaded the California highways, typically with four lanes in each direction. For me to have found a church in Bayfield after only one visit—well, it felt like divine intervention.

As I drove home, I asked for continued guidance and direction in my healing path. I had already made a connection at Namaste to continue with treatments and testing, and I prayed I could conquer this cancer.

29

The Job Hunt

Even though I was not independently wealthy, I was truly enjoying the slow pace of my new life in Colorado, able to take daily walks, attend all of Damiano's soccer practices, and binge watch home improvement and cooking shows such as "Home Town" and "Fall Baking Championship," but I knew this siesta was soon to come to an end. With bills to pay and my career path as a PT to continue, I searched online and joined "Indeed" to help find suitable work. I drove past a few outpatient clinics in the area but didn't get past the front door. For some reason, I had a sense that some were just too sterile for my taste.

One day, while waiting for Damiano to finish his practice, I bumped into Sharon Hunter, a "soccer mom" to whom Julie had previously introduced me. Knowing I was new to the area, she asked me what I did, and I told her I was a physical therapist. She mentioned she taught an exercise class for seniors at the library, and she had heard wonderful things about an outpatient clinic in Bayfield named Pine River PT, ten minutes from my home. She gave me the location and name of the owner, Paula, and encouraged me to walk in and give it a shot. It was getting close to the end of October, and after having a month off, I felt the tug to give it a try.

After compiling a résumé, something I hadn't really needed to do for almost nineteen years since I mostly found jobs through word of mouth in San Diego, I mustered the courage to walk into the Pine River Physical Therapy office and introduce myself. I was greeted by a friendly man named Don, who said he was the husband of the lead PT, Paula Mooney. After explaining that I was new to the area and was a PT looking for part-time work, he looked elated. He said, "You couldn't have come at a more perfect time! One of our PT assistants is leaving for a week's vacation beginning November 11th, and perhaps you could work for us that week. We could see if you're a good fit, and you could decide if you enjoy the work." They asked me to return for a casual interview, and Paula explained that she, like I, had spent many years of her PT career in a skilled rehab setting with the elderly, and decided to venture out on her own and open this clinic upon her patients' requests to keep treating them in an outpatient setting after inpatient rehab. She understood my background and experience level and said she would guide me in the new-to-me setting of outpatient treatments. I couldn't imagine anything more perfect, since I had a slight doubt about my latent, 20-year-old outpatient skill set and whether my techniques would return to me. I could barely contain my excitement! Although outpatient PT was not my typical setting, I had given it a try in Denver almost 20 years prior for a portion of my caseload, mostly treating head-injured or stroke patients and spending the other half of my time doing aqua therapy. Since I had at least dabbled in this realm, I was willing to try it again, refreshing old skills while also gaining completely new ones. Don mentioned that after this trial period, I could perhaps fill in some scheduling gaps during Thanksgiving week and then after the New Year.

November 11th came before I knew it, and although feeling like a fish out of water on the first day, I quickly got into the groove of the treatment style they provided and adapted to the schedule of treating outpatients again. Having predominantly worked in acute care and skilled nursing for the past two decades, there was no true schedule. I would have a list of 8-10 patients to treat on any given day and would find them randomly as they were available, in between IVs, test appointments, wound care treatments, and naps or family visits. Truly enjoying this new patient population, from middle school and high school soccer players and cheerleaders to ranchers who were in their sixties and seventies, I knew Sharon's suggestion was spot on. I had time to get my feet wet, and after that first week took a break and signed up for a few continuing education classes to gain skills and treatment strategies for this new setting.

After that first wonderful week, I got to learn next to Paula, the sole PT in the clinic, who took me under her wing and guided me with patients whose diagnoses or surgeries I had not experienced before. She was patient and incredible at sharing her acquired knowledge with me. I felt confident I could help them in the future as their needs grew.

The month of December arrived, and I noticed a skilled rehab center on my way to Damiano's school. Giving myself an extra fifteen minutes before picking him up, I made my way in and found the rehab department, but the office was empty. I left my number with a staff person, but never received a return call. This building seemed dreary to me anyway, so I wasn't terribly disappointed. I also researched a skilled rehab facility in Durango and decided to walk into their gym. A friendly woman named Gwin greeted me, and I stated that I was a PT new to the area and looking for work. She was ecstatic, saying there was a lack of PTs in the area, and she had planned a one-week vacation during Christmas week. With no one to replace her, she might not be able to take the time off, so she happily gave me a number for the company, and after a call and a phone interview the next day, I was set to begin work the week before Christmas and a few days following.

Everything was falling into place before me, and I felt I could manage both the outpatient setting and this and have a change of pace. Later, I found out a rehab facility just so happened to need a PT two times a week beginning in January to cover a three-month sabbatical for an employee. Don and Paula had mentioned they may need me three times a week starting sometime in January, so the puzzle pieces were fitting together perfectly. This balance would be great, where I could do work familiar to me for a few days and work that challenged me the rest of the week. I could take a deep breath, knowing I had found a way to enjoy my career with a varied schedule.

30

✤

Added Confirmation

One weekend, when Damiano had a soccer tournament followed by a soccer party at a pizza place in Farmington, New
Mexico, I decided to make the one-hour trip. Julie was there,
of course—she rarely missed a soccer game—and she introduced me to
more of the soccer parents. Since I knew Sharon Hunter, I noticed her at
the soccer party and asked if I could join her in her booth. She welcomed
me and introduced me to her husband and her son, Lane, the goalie, one
of Damiano's favorite friends on the team.

After telling her I was now working at Paula's clinic, I reiterated how
thankful I was that she had led me there, as it was truly a wonderful fit
for me. As we dove deeper into conversation, the topic of health came up.
She mentioned she had recovered from a battle with cancer and had been
treated naturally by a wonderful doctor. Eager to hear who treated her, she
said she went to Namaste and Nasha Winters had been her practitioner.
I was stunned. The very same clinician I had been following on the internet and whose interviews I watched had treated Sharon! What a small
world—I felt confirmation I was getting treatment at the right clinic.
What were the chances? Nasha Winters and Namaste could have been
anywhere in the US, and I had now found her and befriended one of her

clients in my new hometown! She explained that Nasha had gone on to write books and was speaking internationally about cancer healing, but, with nothing but wonderful things to say about Nasha and her Durango clinic, I would continue in Sharon's footsteps and seek that same care.

Since January had already arrived, I knew it was time to keep up with my recommended MRI and scheduled a trip to Denver. Paula and Don were incredibly supportive and told me to schedule it whenever it was needed, and to take my time and not rush back. For me, this could be an adventure mixed with a reunion of prior coworkers and friends, and amazingly, I was able to organize meetings with six friends while there. I first traveled to Boulder to visit my friend Susie LeFebevre from PT school in Philadelphia, who had originally inspired me to move to Colorado. We took walks near a small lake in the cold, winter temperatures, and she encouraged me on my path to healing, mentioning that she and her daughter were also making dietary changes due to sensitivities to gluten. This was a popular topic now, and almost everyone seemed educated in it, but when I was first struggling a few decades prior with health issues, traditional doctors thought people like me who complained of stomach or headaches from foods as being "all in our heads."

One incredible reunion was with my friend Nancy Corson, whom I had not seen since we both adopted our sons, almost twenty years prior. We had been in a required adoption class together, and after finding out she was an occupational therapist, we formed an unspoken bond with a strong faith and a common career path that reflected our personalities as caregivers. Meeting with her in Littleton for a cup of tea was certainly fitting since it was frigid outside. She didn't know why I was in Denver, but I shared my cancer story and why I had opted not to do surgery as of yet. I conveyed how I felt God was really speaking to me about seeking a natural path, and she mentioned a friend she knew who was battling cancer, so I shared my advice that cancer feeds on sugar, not mainstream knowledge at the time.

The following day, I met with friends Paula Cahill and Lauren Molina, also PTs who I'd met at Mercy Medical Center, a friendly, little hospital that sadly had been razed, leaving all who worked there jobless. These women were dynamic and knowledgeable in many areas, and though they questioned why I was seeking a non-traditional path, they bolstered me with support and enthusiasm and agreed to meet at a restaurant that would support my dietary limitations. We had a great time reminiscing about old friends and times we shared in our twenties in downtown Denver's Larimer Square, and the fated night that Paula and I met her husband-to-be, Matt, while playing pool at the Wynkoop Brewery—something I was not particularly adept at but that Paula seemed to master that night. This skill, and the confidence and shine in her eyes, led her to this man, whom I just happened to bump into the next morning at breakfast with a friend. I made sure to get his number for Paula, and I assured him that she may have a fancy for him—and the rest is history.

My friend Karin Zimmerman, also a Mercy alum, who was hired as a PT perhaps a month after me at our ripe age of twenty-four, housed me for two nights, and filled me with wonderful meals and memories. We took walks and she shared stories of her daughter Kailey's new passion for rescuing dogs. One story in particular struck me about a dog named Rudy who had been so neglected, his collar had grown into his skin, and the vets had to surgically remove it. He was also malnourished, and Kailey and her fellow sorority sisters at Auburn had to nurse him back to health. This was amazing to me to hear these young students were choosing such humanitarian acts rather than the "party scene" so common on college campuses. Karin was extremely supportive of me during this time and welcomed me to come back as many times as I needed during my journey.

Finally, January 14 arrived, the day my MRI was scheduled and a day I was anticipating. I felt this day would be telling—letting me know if I had made a mistake or confirming that I could heal without surgery. I had time to meet my friend Nicki Shier, an occupational therapist and

Mercy Medical Center alum, and a frequent part of the pack that used to socialize together on many weekend nights in Denver in our twenties. Driving down I-25 to meet Nicki, I got a phone call that surprised and filled my heart. Chris Bernard, the senior pastor from Life Church, wanted to say a prayer with me before my test. I was shocked that he would take time out of his busy schedule to call and encourage me, speaking words of healing over me that would come from God alone. As I was driving, I felt confident that the test would go well and was hopeful for the results. My time with Nicki was wonderful, and we shared updates about our children, one whom she had naturally and one she adopted. Since children who are adopted sometimes have similar learning or emotional challenges, we encouraged each other through the ups and downs. She also said a prayer for me before my MRI, and I entered the facility in Englewood, Colorado, with confidence and peace. The nurse administering the IV asked me if I needed to take anything for anxiety, and I responded that this wasn't necessary. She offered me a variety of music choices, something I realized was pointless, since the rattling sounds of the magnets dwarfed any sound the music was making. As I was lying face down on the table, I imagined a native tribe in some faraway land beating on drums or other instruments. The nurse informed me that if I wasn't really still, they may have to cancel the test and re-administer it at a later time. Knowing this was not an option for me, I remained immobile, like a mannequin in a store window, hesitant to even breathe. After the forty-five-minute test, the IV that provided the contrast dye to reveal the areas needing to be inspected was removed from my arm. I left the facility at dusk and got on my way for the nearly six-hour drive home through the mountains. Knowing this wasn't the wisest decision, my stubborn nature compelled me to get home and back to work. Deer and other wildlife were more active at night and often crossed the roads, causing accidents, and rogue storms were common at 10,000 feet on Wolf Creek Pass, but I pressed on. A few days later, I received a call from the nurse practitioner at the MRI center, telling me that the tumor was still there, but the size of it had reduced from 1 to 0.8 centimeters, a reduction of 2 millimeters. At first, I must admit, this news was disappointing. Of course, there was a part of me that wished I would be that rare person whose tumor disappeared. After all, I had done at least twelve, if not fourteen, vitamin C IV infusions for several hours at a time, took many recommended supplements, and hadn't eaten any sugar over the holidays. But reflecting on the fact that the tumor had shrunk and not grown in six months, I felt I could keep on keeping on. New ideas and diets flashed through my mind, and I was determined to keep researching cancer and healing methods. Would I need to surrender and get the mastectomy, or would I be one of the few and fortunate ones to avoid this invasive approach? Only time would tell.

31

The Dark Pandemic

Who would have thought that with whispers of people in China having a deadly virus, the entire world was headed for the worst pandemic since the bubonic plague, forcing us into a lockdown? Lukas enlisted in the Marines and started boot camp in Point Loma, California, on December 15, 2019. Interestingly, this was the same date I met him as a two-year-old at his orphanage, a memory branded in my mind since leaving the comforts of Denver for a journey to Romania ten days before Christmas of 1997. Since the day he entered boot camp, I'd written to him weekly, sometimes several times a week. He had also written me letters indicating this was the biggest mental challenge he or perhaps anyone could overcome. Not knowing how important the graduation ceremony was to Lukas, or any Marine, I mentioned to my friend Melanie Turner, whose husband was a retired Marine Corps helicopter pilot, that I may not be able to travel to the event. She countered with an affirmative response. "Kristi, you absolutely should not miss graduation. This ceremony is so important to the men who have been in boot camp, separated from all outside communication and enduring the most emotionally, physically, and mentally challenging time in their lives. It is something you need to attend."

Thankful for her direct guidance and for explaining to me something I was truly naive about, I asked Paula and Don the next day for several days off to afford myself the chance to attend his graduation event. Unfortunately, on the very last day of February 2020, I felt a tickle in my throat and was experiencing labored breathing, causing me to wheeze. Working closely amongst patients who traveled all over the US, I was a prime candidate for the spread of the virus. Not suspecting anything that weekend since I was not feverish, and didn't have congestion or a sore throat, I wondered why my breathing was so shallow and raspy. For two nights, I could barely get a breath, but hospitals on the news were advising to avoid ERs as long as possible and try to stay home as they were beginning to become flooded with those struck by the suffocating effects of COVID-19.

Thankfully, I had a few days off during the period when I would be a known spreader of the virus, and I remained solitary and away from every soul possible. One night, desperately struggling to get air, I looked for an inhaler in my medicine cabinet with no luck and considered heading to the ER. Suddenly, I thought of my friend and health coach, Monica Pelle, who told me of a "flu bomb" mixture of essential oils to use for flu symptoms or difficulty breathing. After walking in the dark into my office, I read her instructions. In a small amount of water, combine two drops each of lavender, peppermint, and lemon essential oils and drink it. WOW, the results were astounding! I instantly felt my airway open, allowing deeper, although still shallow breaths, permitting me to sleep—something that had been eluding me. Also intriguing was that I was able to avoid the use of a steroid inhaler that had side effects I wanted to avoid, and all thanks to that conversation I'd had with Monica that fall day about the healing nature of oils!

My symptoms of labored breathing improved, but then those of fever, body aches, and head congestion hit and before I knew it, the raspy sounds of my breath when I exhaled or inhaled indicated I might have pneumonia or at least bronchitis. I suspected I was one of the first people with COVID in the county, but by the time I felt strong enough to go to the county fairgrounds for testing, they turned me away, saying I didn't have the symptoms that qualified me for the test. Lukas's graduation was slowly getting closer, and I would need to fly. I would be required to wear a mask, and I hoped by then my symptoms would dissipate so I wouldn't be a super-spreader of the virus, or whatever I had.

The date of March 12 arrived, and, donning my mask, I boarded the plane, with all other passengers doing the same. I kept my lozenges on hand, dare a cough be triggered and anyone spew hateful stares my way. Of course, as fate would have it, there was a rogue storm striking Phoenix of all places, so my plane was delayed, and when I finally made it there, I had missed my connecting flight to San Diego. The graduation was the next morning, and sweat beaded on my forehead as I conjured up images of missing his ceremony. Fortunately, after spending the night in Phoenix, I was able to catch the first flight out, and Erica—who would be attending his graduation ceremony with me—was able to get me to the event by 7:00 a.m. We were one of the first cars through the gate, and to say I was amazed at the turnout would be an understatement. After passing through security and finding our way into a massive indoor auditorium, we joined hundreds of other parents and families from West of the Mississippi for what we hoped would be a wonderful celebration for Lukas and the many other brave men's accomplishments. My parents and husband had not yet arrived but called to say they were waiting at the entrance gate. While trying to prevent any coughing with my lozenges in use, a person of authority approached the stage and abruptly announced they had just received word from Marine headquarters that this Marine graduation would be canceled. It was March 13, the day it was declared by our government that COVID-19 was a national pandemic. None of us could know the season of hysteria and despair we were about to enter.

Lukas recalls that he and his battalion, India company, were running perhaps the first of three miles in the "Motto" run, or motivational run, that concluded their physical vigor—the first time we as families would see them as they ran into the stadium, after thirteen weeks of training. Suddenly, during a torrential downpour, they were ordered to a halt. Knowing they would never be ordered to stop due to any amount of rain, they all thought they had done something wrong. Instead, they were informed they would not be performing their drills, would not have a ceremony, and would not see their families that day—something for which they had been longing for months. The military had to organize a system for them to be picked up the following day, and none of us knew just what that was at that time. Fiercely disappointed, they all returned to their barracks and awaited direction.

The following day, we were notified to come to the military base in Point Loma and, remaining in our cars, look for a booth labeled with the last initial of our sons' names. My dad and I made our way to the base and inched along as we saw many troops waiting for their families under beige tents. When we pulled up to the letter "W," the sergeant called Lukas's name and directed him toward our car, but I opened the window and said to the man, "That is not my son," since he had gained perhaps twenty-five pounds and looked more "beefy" and muscular than I was accustomed to seeing him. The sergeant responded coldly, "Ma'am, this is certainly your son," and I noticed a quizzical look on Lukas's face as if to say, "My own mom doesn't even recognize me." Not permitted to get out of our cars due to pandemic rules, Lukas loaded his backpack into the trunk and hopped in the back seat of the car. Only then did I recognize those deep, dark, surveying eyes. Embarrassed that I had not recognized him, I told him I was sorry, but he looked so different, and he agreed that those thirteen weeks had changed him like he never imagined it could. This would be more obvious when we were at home, but for the time being, we congratulated him and told him how proud we were of him to have completed boot camp and accomplished what many could not—the honor of becoming a Marine.

Shortly after arriving home, those physical changes became really apparent. For instance, when talking to me, Tim, and my dad in the living room, he stood at attention, as if one of us were about to scold him for slouching. I joked with him, "Lukas, you can relax. I'm not going to ask you to do any push-ups or sit-ups." He commented that he wasn't aware he was standing that way and was so used to the everyday formal posture, he would have to re-learn how to be a civilian.

We had a wonderful celebration and welcome home party for him with our family, Erica and Jerome, his childhood mentor Jesse Almanza, childhood friend Jesse Jonhson, close friend Dahlia, and his "great godparents," Carol and John Groseth. He looked radiant, a look of humble pride across his face, if there is such a thing. Despite the many learning challenges and physical ailments he had battled all his life, he was grateful, as were all of us, that he had completed such an arduous goal. We ate all of his favorite foods and desserts, including the most decadent chocolate cake, even though he wasn't such a sweets lover.

Savoring every minute with him, since he had to return to Camp Pendleton for the School of Infantry in ten days, we enjoyed good conversation, rest, and rejuvenation. Needing to return to Colorado for work, my parents were going to take him back to his assignment, and I would persist in my attempts to shrink the cancer inside of me.

During that pandemic season, however, everyone's elective medical appointments and tests were being pushed back, so when it came time for my six-month follow-up in July, I was informed it would be a few more months before I would be able to get the MRI I needed. This was not a surprise since people with more dire or emergent issues were triaged as more necessary, and even some of my patients were expressing frustration at having surgeries delayed several months. Knowing this, I continued my vegan diet with no sugar, confident that when the day came for testing, my tumor would respond accordingly.

Back in the Durango area, I went to Julie's house often since her husband was in Telluride for work and Tim was in San Diego completing the build of his sister's home. Restaurants weren't open, but food carts were, and being mega-fans of the Eleventh Street food carts, we ordered Thai food from one of them perhaps twice a week. They had vegan dishes compatible with my diet, and Tatiana, Damiano, and Julie all encouraged me to stick to my diet to conquer that cancer. Julie was pivotal in convincing me to "eat clean" and convicted me in an incredibly sisterly way if I were tempted to "cheat" on my eating plan. I can almost hear her now if I ever reached for a chocolate chip cookie, saying, "Kristi, you just have to do this for a season. You can do this." Being an amazing cook herself, at my beck and call, she offered to sauté purple cabbage with garlic and vinegar or whatever other healthy concoctions she could whip up to help me enjoy the tastes that went along with this pure foods diet.

Being limited in all aspects of the entertainment realm, Tatiana and I discovered a bent toward puzzles, and searching the game section in Walmart, found that every other family in Southwest Colorado must also be trying to occupy their time with puzzles, as often the shelves would be wiped bare. Since I worked twice a week in Pagosa Springs, which was more remote than Durango, I would hit their Walmart and often find a great 500-piece puzzle. But once out of desperation, with no engaging material available, I noticed a puzzle containing 1,000 pieces sitting on top of a dresser in my patient's room. Oddly, it had sat there untouched for months, and, after asking the activities director if I could borrow it, she happily said yes. We both knew that residents of this building were often challenged with ten to twenty-piece, rudimentary puzzles, and this puzzle was much too advanced. I promised to put it in a five-day isolation period and sanitize it before bringing it back. It ended up being the most frustrating one "Tati" and I tackled, with far too many white, nondescript clouds or blue sky, making it nearly impossible to look for patterns or color differences that were typically used to help put puzzles together, but one we finished with gratitude. Knowing that, any guilt I might have had for taking it soon vanished, as it would have been torture for any of my patients with dementia to conquer.

32

Unexpected Move

My parents were feeling cooped up in their home in San Diego during the pandemic. Some of their closest friends moved away to the Carolinas or to Northern California. Since my dad's golf buddies were dwindling, and he wanted to experience Damiano's and Tatiana's soccer adventures up close and personal rather than virtually, he coaxed my mom into selling their home and moving in with us. Julie had now moved to Durango as well, and Tatiana had left her high school in Telluride and was in Durango too, so they didn't see the point in spending a few more years in San Diego separated from all of us. My mom, who was reluctant and unconvinced that she was ready to leave her posse of friends, finally acquiesced to the idea since their church was closed due to the pandemic, limiting many of her gatherings that were focused around the church.

My dad had made a bold proclamation at the dinner table in San Diego before Tim and I moved that he wanted to join us immediately, and when we were hunting for homes, we took my mom with us to find something that would suit all of us, with separate living spaces for them and us so they could "age in place" rather than going to a senior living facility when reaching the golden years. Since I had nineteen years of firsthand experience working in facilities for the elderly and heard the prolific complaints about staff shortages and such from the residents living there, I figured this solution would be best for our family. Our home was ready for my parents whenever they were ready. We hadn't anticipated them coming for perhaps another five years, but the isolation imposed by the pandemic sped up their timeline, and here they came. I was looking forward to this again, since for years as a single mom, I lived with my parents as I raised Lukas, and we got along famously. I would again have the chance to bond with my dad while we watched sports, as we had since I was a child. My mom and I would be able to shop together, go to church together, and talk about everything like we always did.

Thankfully, Tim was wrapping up the home build for his sister and finishing work projects for Erica and Jerome, and would finally be able to join me in Colorado the first week in May. My parents would follow in the early summer. They weren't sure how long it would take to sell their home, but we all thought it wouldn't take long.

My friend Chrissy Stone and her husband Steve listed the home, and perhaps seven days later, it was sold, making their move a reality sooner than my mom had hoped but not soon enough for my dad. Unfortunately, one day, while in the hallway of her San Diego home, about to begin packing, my mom spun around quickly while the Birkenstocks she was wearing did not and lost her balance, striking her trunk on the door jam and slithering her way to the floor with instant and debilitating pain. Having fractured several ribs, that posse of friends she loved so much came to her rescue, packed up my parents' entire home, and soon got them on their way to all of us, and their new home in Durango.

33

Testing Time & Reunion

T
he MRI center informed me that my position in the queue had finally come, and an appointment for my follow-up was available in early October. Even though I needed to travel to Denver to keep monitoring my tumor, I decided I needed to keep a "cup half full" attitude and turn it into reunion time with my Denver comrades. I contacted the bunch, including Karin Zimmerman, Paula Cahill, Lauren Molina, and Nicki Shier, and all of us were able to gather at one of our favorite spots from years-gone-by at the Wash Park Grille (short for Washington Park). Everyone was so thankful to be able to get together again, after being in what felt like family confinement to many. Since I lived in a rural region and had only one neighbor at the time, I could freely take my daily walks unmasked (I don't think the deer or other wildlife were "social distancing"), whereas all my city friends were more limited in their ability to exercise or socialize. We reminisced about the good old days, and updated one another on what our lives and our kids' lives were filled with, whether now attending college or playing soccer or lacrosse for this school or that.

Able to also travel to Boulder to see Susie Lefebvre, she encouraged me to stay on my diet by making a to-die-for, gluten-free, vegan salad with quinoa. We also had time to go for a walk and to soak in the beauty near the Flatirons. These were a series of hills with jutting and jagged surfaces but resembled an iron if looking at them from a certain angle.

Karin Zimmerman housed me for most of the trip, and we talked about our work. I expressed that the pace of my work in the outpatient clinic was manageable, but having sleep deficits that had plagued me my entire life, and I was not getting any younger, I was starting to feel wiped out at the end of the day. I could keep my momentum for my patients, and once the day was over, close to 6:00 p.m., my energy store was empty, and the best dinner my husband could hope for was one cooked by my mom or from the local Chinese restaurant, Hong's Garden.

Karin encouraged me to listen to my body and to pay attention to the warning signs of fatigue and difficulty sleeping. She knew me well and commented that our shared strong work ethic, like many in our generation, was a good thing, but it also could work to my detriment. With compassion and understanding, she gently suggested that if my workload was too great for my current situation, I had a choice to walk away, and didn't need to please others over my own health needs. Perhaps it is a character trait of people who work in health care—they seem to be the worst at taking care of themselves until the rubber meets the road, so to speak. I thanked her for her honesty and her advice, and as we meandered through her neighborhood on a chilly but brilliant day, a feeling began to brew in me to begin to slow down my pace, but I wasn't quite ready to listen to that voice yet.

Driving home from Denver, in figurative and literal valleys lined with plots of land set aside for farming, I passed cows and empty fields that were past their harvest, and wondered what the results of the test would show. Sooner than I imagined, early the following week, I got a call from the nurse at the MRI center stating that the tumor was still there, it had not yet disappeared as I had hoped, and was back to its original size at one cm. Of course, the wind was taken out of my sails, but being that it remained status quo, I still did not feel the urgency for a mastectomy. Time was still on my side. Remembering the words of Christine's oncologist, who told her she could potentially wait three years before being concerned about surgery with a 1.5-centimeter mass, I wanted to forge ahead and figure out this path to natural healing.

34

Words of Truth and Beauty

H as anyone experienced a season of their life during which they received unsolicited advice? Cancer also falls in this category, and, in my case, I received books from friends about cancer that I hadn't asked for but were gifts from heaven. They were poignant, humorous, and engaging. Going out on a limb here, if you the reader are adverse to reading about a season of adversity you are going through such as, "How to navigate as a newly single woman after divorce," that a friend sent you, dive in, absorb it, and soak it in rather than being secretly irritated that someone not in your shoes thinks they know better about what you're battling. Even though they don't know, chances are you will glean a nugget of encouragement or insight that you may not otherwise have received if you can be an open vessel and prepared for the love your friend wants to share with you.

The first to arrive in the mail was from my dear friend Alexandra, titled *Cancer, My Love* by Mioara Grigore. This memoir particularly struck a chord with me because the author was from Romania. Since I spent six months there, sprinkled throughout each season of the year while working at an orphanage in a more than remote town in Transylvania, I resonated with her in a cultural and spiritual way. Her writing, which exposed her cancer battle, truly pierced my soul with vulnerability and an utter rawness that reflected a rare humility. Describing herself as a somewhat self-righteous religion teacher and oddly wanting to impress a despised fellow colleague, she, unfortunately, tumbled down a flight of stairs in a skirt and high heels to the feet of this red-haired man. Since he was a professed atheist, she was determined to hate every inch of him, but instead fell madly in love with him, had five children, one with Down's syndrome, and then was diagnosed with breast cancer that was ravaging through her body. Trying every remedy known to man—something that had me chuckling since I was doing just that—she went on a quest to cure cancer by eating herbs and veggies, only to resort to royally binging on strips of bacon when she didn't receive the results of shrinkage for which she had hoped. Believing in her heart of hearts that she would heal, she left the reader cheering her on until it was clear she would succumb to the disease and leave behind her five beautiful children in the devastated hands of Viorel, the love of her life. While hiking to the top of Caraiman Peak in the Bucegi Mountains at an altitude of 7,516 feet with her family—with stage IV cancer that had spread from her breast to her liver and lungs—she collapsed on a pile of large boulders along the way. Since she felt as though she had no air left in her lungs, and may truly have had very little, three of her children pushed her from behind, and two pulled her by her left hand, while Viorel pulled her by her right hand toward the top. They willed her to do what she otherwise would not have been able to accomplish—reach Heroes' Cross at the very pinnacle, a cross she said, "Waited for me patiently, as it had waited for me all my life."[10]

While reading about her hike to the top, I was literally weeping, tears streaming down my cheeks, with sadness that her children would lose their mother and her husband his passionate love, but also an indescribable joy that she felt as she awaited meeting her God.

---

[10] Mioara Grigore, *Cancer, My Love* (Platina, CA: St. Heron of Alaska Brotherhood, 2008), 216.

The words spoken during an interview before her passing still penetrate my core, as she boldly said, "There are saints among us. These people have prolonged my life through their love. And so, I live in almost cosmic wonder—how is it that I haven't died yet? According to oncology, the cancer scattered in my lungs and liver should have taken over, devastating me completely. However, it seems that the love of these people has kept my metastases stagnant. I believe the miracle God gave me of encountering them has greatly superseded the miracle of physical healing."[11] This book changed my perspective during my journey, and without it, I may have become self-focused on my healing rather than seeing what others were doing for me through their encouragement, and what I could still do for others during my battle.

One evening, alone at home, I received a phone call from my cousin, Lara Grady, wondering whether I would mind if she sent me a book written by the pastor of her church. She was already gracious enough to ask me, and with her ever-gentle spirit, said the book had touched her heart, and thought it would mine. What thoughtfulness to call and ask if I would mind if she sent an inspirational book to me! Assuring her I would welcome it, several days later, it arrived in the mail. Not taking a minute to let it gather dust on a shelf, I delved into the pages of *Gold in the Road: Through the Cancer Storm with Jesus Christ,* written by Reverend Cathie Young. In this book, I not only found nuggets of gold but also other gemstones of love and peace and joy. During Cathie's personal journey with aggressive breast cancer, requiring bilateral mastectomies, radiation, and debilitating chemotherapy, she witnessed to everyone she encountered along the way about the God she loved. I recall that even while undergoing radiation, minutes after or before her treatment, she prayed with the radiation tech, showing selflessness and sharing God's love while receiving treatments that would later cause her burning pain. Also, while being infused with chemotherapy, she was a bright light to everyone in the room going through

---

[11] Grigore, *Cancer, My Love*, 252–253.

their own treatments. The love and joy she shared was truly humbling, and to this day, she has retired from her position as pastor at Orange County Church, where my cousin met her, and leads a cancer support group, allowing those who suffer and who are battling cancer to get the emotional encouragement they need to endure the battle. And to think my dear cousin Lara was hesitant to send it or even to ask, not wanting to offend me, perhaps. When I think of this, I remember those fleeting thoughts I had during the first few weeks after my diagnosis of stage zero cancer, when people wanted to offer advice, and I may have shrugged it off internally. Thinking back to this, I would have been a fool not to receive what others thought would be of benefit to me. This book continues to remind me of the selfless approach Cathie took during her battle. Instead, she fought side by side with others every step of the way.

My friend, Sue Scott, precious to me due to the bond we shared as adoptive mothers, also excitedly asked me if she could send me a book written by her friend, who had battled cancer. Her enthusiasm for the book was palpable, and I readily agreed. I devoured this book as Tim and I took a trip to Santa Fe, New Mexico, both to enjoy the beauty of the land, get away for a few days, and to see what the consignment shops friends had recommended to us had to offer. The book, titled *Chemo P!ssed Me Off: A Breast Cancer Roadmap: Navigating with Faith, Gratitude, and a Little Bit of Attitude* and written by Carol Wyllie, allowed me to be more human during my experience. She expressed raw emotions I tended to keep buried inside, and raw irritation toward some, if not most, of her doctors, that I would typically word more conservatively. But her approach of "let it all out" was truly freeing. She had a similar stage zero and DCIS cancer and chose a radical approach, but also entertained and employed some alternative measures, and this was also inspiring to see. Her use of humor was otherworldly. I recall a comment she made to her general surgeon when she was explaining why she was declining chemotherapy at the time, and she assured him she was not going to travel to a third-world country to drink shark urine. Remembering some of the odd concoctions I used to try to keep my cancer at bay, I had to laugh out loud, and this laughter in and of itself was therapeutic.

The author emphasized how her medical team would at times forget the little things since they were commonly on autopilot during their jobs. During one of nearly thirty radiation treatments, tears were streaming down her cheeks as she truly was resistant to the procedure, and even though she had just been told to not move her arms, head, or any part of her body—and her nurse was aware of that—he thoughtfully brought her a tissue to wipe her tears and placed it in her hand; but since she was immobilized she was unable to use it. Note to self: Even when overwhelmed at work or in any atmosphere, if trying to be compassionate and caring, think through everything so you don't leave someone who is paralyzed with a tissue they can't use. Go the extra mile and wipe the tears from their cheeks.

During an appointment with her radiologist, who discussed the effects of radiation on her already reconstructed implant from her mastectomy, the doctor informed her that the radiation could tighten the area around her implant and cause the breast to look disfigured. Because the radiated skin could take a year to heal, and at times the skin remained tough, people might want to choose to have reconstruction on their unaffected breast so it would match. Her internal dialogue thought, "Whoa, Whoa—wait!" and then stated to the doctor, "Excuse me for being frank, but you're telling me that my implant may end up looking more like an earring instead of a boob, and the medical world's solution to that is to give me another earring? You have gotta be kidding me!" Since these were men talking to her, she thought to herself that she would prefer a woman and added her motto, "No uterus, no opinion."[12] Needless to say, her quick wit and willingness to be upfront and vulnerable

---

[12] Carol M. Wyllie, *Chemo P!ssed Me Off: A Breast Cancer Road Map: Navigating with Faith, Gratitude, and a Little Bit of Attitude* (Dub Press, 2012), 104–105.

with the doctors were refreshing to me since I typically held everything in, allowing things to brew for years rather than expressing it, letting it out, and letting go, as she did.

She also riddled her story with Bible verses, including one from the Proverbs. "Where there is strife there is pride, but wisdom is found in those who take advice. Whoever scorns instruction will pay for it, but whoever respects a command is rewarded. The teaching of the wise is a fountain of life, turning a person from the snares of death" (Proverbs 13:10, 13–14, NIV). How true this was. If I had been resistant to reading this, I would have missed out on many belly laughs and much-needed permission to release my emotions, along with verses that spoke to my soul.

Tim ordered me several books from a science-based perspective that will be discussed later in this book, but finally, as far as non-scientific books people gave me, one was unexpected and came at the right time. My friends, chiropractors Donna and Tom Stuebe, both treated Lukas and me and also became dear friends of the entire family. They were amazing people, and invited Tim, Lukas and me to join them when they served the homeless in downtown San Diego near Petco Park. We would all travel downtown, meeting people and handing out burritos Donna made, and chocolate chip cookies I had made. This brings to mind a memorable moment I feel must be mentioned. Lukas could recall every name of every homeless person with whom we made a significant connection, and one named Leroy came up excitedly to me to receive his sandwich bag filled with two cookies. He and the others knew that they only received one bag per person. Later in the evening, as Lukas and I came around the block, Leroy approached me again and said, "I have a word from the Lord for you." Instantly, I was mesmerized and could barely wait to hear what God had spoken to him for me. Would it be that I would be cancer-free for the rest of my life, or be able to adopt five more kids and live happily ever after? He developed a serious look on his face and said, "God wants to tell you to give me two more cookies." I bent over in hysterics while he was grinning from ear to ear. I couldn't resist and went against my one bag per person policy and gave him another bag of chocolate chip cookies as he reached out to receive them with a smile.

Now back to the Stuebe's. Donna had been diagnosed with an ailment and was traveling to the area to see a local practitioner, and asked if her sister, Mindy Milligan, could join them. We happily invited her to stay with us, especially since they lived sixteen hours apart. Since I was in Durango, she was only five to six hours away, and they could have a reunion. After we had a wonderful time with Mindy, sharing meals and board games and late-night talks, she offered to send me a book written by her neighbor, titled *Fear Less, Love More: What to Do When the Unexpected Happens*, written by Dr. Kathryn Haber. Suffering the unimaginable and the tremendous loss of her father, mother, sister, and brother to cancer, she herself was diagnosed with cancer while raising three children under the age of three, including six-month-old twins. A clinical psychologist by trade, she was a professed agnostic prior to her diagnosis and did not entertain the thought of God until the time when she was told she had cancer. A few weeks after her diagnosis, with fear and panic raging through her mind and body, she collapsed on the floor of her bathroom and called out to God, asking for strength and praying for him to spare her life, allow her children to grow up with a mother, and for her husband not to be left without his wife. She hadn't prayed since she'd said the Lord's Prayer as a child, and now she found herself begging for help. After several minutes, a peace and calm swept over her, her breathing calmed, and she felt so much lighter, she wondered if this could be God answering her prayers. She then walked through her cancer battle, not from a stance of defeat, but victory. She learned to choose love and compassion rather than criticism and judgment, and faith, prayer, and vulnerability over fear to help battle any defeating circumstance or illness.[13]

---

[13] Dr. Kathryn Haber, *Love More: What to Do When the Unexpected Happens: Five Daily Choices* (Virginia: Koehler Books, 2020).

The words of wisdom from these four cancer survivors were invaluable, and I am thankful I welcomed them into my life during my own cancer journey. Since it is proven that stress—which would include fear—is a factor in the cause of some cancers, specifically breast cancer, I knew I benefited from every page I read in these four books, reflecting a spirit of faith that bolstered healing or the ability to weather the storm of the disease. I will be forever grateful for all my friends who had the instinct to share these books with me and the follow-through to send them to me. If anyone in your circle invites you to do the same, accept the invitation. The answer to some of your questions in your healing path may just rest in the words between the pages.

35

※

The Uncertain Road to Healing

Feelings of doubt began to mount within me. Questioning all the diets and methods I had tried, my tumor remained as it had begun, and this fact was plaguing me. I continued to adhere to a vegan diet up to the time of my next MRI in Denver that following April. Housed and welcomed again by my friends Susie Lefebvre and Karin Zimmerman in Boulder and Denver, respectively, I could sense their concern that mirrored mine that perhaps if the results did not make a drastic change, I would need to consider the dreaded surgery I was trying to avoid. Although they both gave me nothing but the utmost support and understanding, the hope I had at the onset was beginning to wane like the moon after its fullest state. Did I really hear God's voice telling me not to do the surgery? Maybe that was just because of that insensitive surgeon who referred to me as "one of those, someone who was vain and not ready to let go of my body part." I suppose she thought it was a worthless appendage, ready to be whacked off at the slightest hint of cancer, or the suspicion thereof. For me, this was not a simple decision, most likely due to my line of work, which included post-mastectomy care. Treating patients who suffered from chest and back pain and also lymphedema, or swelling in the arm of the surgical site that lasted indefinitely, I was truly torn with this decision. Time was still on my side, but the clock was ticking, and I was only allowing myself until the end of 2022 to toy around with this disease that could permeate my being. With my science-minded background, I was determined to not let this tumor metastasize. The surgery would surely happen by then, and that surgeon could no longer refer to me as "one of those."

Not feeling optimal and somewhat listless on the vegan diet, I made the pilgrimage to the Denver area, but this time had the MRI done in Golden, just after having lunch with my "godsister," Deborah Simon. She—who I could tell was worried beyond measure that I was waiting too long—was honest with me and said she would pray for me and understood what I was doing, but also made me promise I would have the surgery if I needed it. Of course, giving her my promise, I hoped it wouldn't come to that. Shortly after making my way home, while near the town of Del Norte, I received the call that the tumor was actually expanding and was now 1.3 centimeters in size. As I climbed Wolf Creek Pass, with tears streaming down my cheeks as big as the raindrops that fell on the mountain's peak, a song came on the radio by Lauren Daigle called "Trust in You," which talked about being weary and needing rest, but also that God was the king of the fight. Could I trust him? I knew in my soul the answer was yes, but maybe his answer wasn't going to look the way I wanted it to. With rain pelting my windshield, I wondered what the answer would be. Time was ticking, and the bomb felt like it was getting that much closer to exploding.

At home, I shared the unfortunate news with Tim, and I told him I wanted to try everything possible and learn everything possible to heal naturally, and only then would I surrender. He got on the computer that minute and ordered three books for me: *How to Starve Cancer* by Jane McLelland, *I Cure Cancer* by Ian Jackson, and *The Stengler Cancer-Reversing Protocol* by Dr. Mark Stengler, NMD, from the Encinitas clinic where I'd started my intravenous vitamin C treatments. Once they arrived, I tore through the first by Jane McLelland page by page, written ironically by a physical therapist who shared my passion for trying to figure out how to heal. She had stage IV cancer and was given little hope of survival, and one gem of information I recall was that since she learned that cancer fed on sugar, she asked her doctor to give her the drug Metformin, typically used for diabetics to control their blood sugar. She also figured out very complex chemistry solutions that even her oncologists had to study to decipher, but after understanding what she was intending, she used these formulas along with a diet free of sugar, and she outlived their prognosis for her to die in six months, living fourteen years and counting, long enough to write her story. This bolstered my confidence and gave me an ounce of courage, if not more, to keep trying this route. The Stengler-based protocol highlighted movement and its ability to reduce a breast cancer patient's risk of dying from the disease by 40 percent with only a brisk, thirty-minute walk several times a week, according to one study.[14] Who was out on a walk daily, rain or shine? Me! It also encouraged daily use of chamomile tea or chamomile supplements since it contains a substance called apigenin that, in several experiments with breast cancer cells, corrected the defect in cancer cells, allowing them to live longer than other cells. I couldn't complain about drinking a cup or two daily, while also drinking green tea.[15]

The last book about curing cancer was still on the shelf as I employed some of the strategies of the first two. It would come, perhaps at the intended time.

---

[14] Stengler, *The Stengler*, 80.

[15] Stengler, *The Stengler*, 29.

36

Unorthodox Methods—a Cure
or a Curse?

C all me crazy, but at this point, I was willing to try everything and anything to cure my cancer. Receiving a well-meaning call from my beloved brother-in-law, Russell Bitter, he excitedly said, "Kristi, I have something I need you to try. I heard about it and really think it could help, and I think it is based on science and has had positive results for cancer patients." Asking him to share what it was, he replied, "It includes cottage cheese mixed with flaxseed oil. Let's pray that it helps." He mentioned a verse I knew from Matthew that said where two or more are gathered in Jesus' name,[16] he is there among us, and I thanked him for his advice, hung up the phone, and literally drove to the store to get cottage cheese and flaxseed oil. Now, I didn't really like cottage cheese and hadn't eaten it since my pregnancy with twins years earlier, when it was the only thing I could stomach, while I craved absolutely nothing and was nauseated every minute of every day. It was the only thing I could manage during those nine months, and I hadn't eaten it before or since, but I was

---

[16] Matthew 18:20

willing to give it a try. I researched the cottage cheese and flaxseed oil combo and its effects on cancer, and lo and behold, a well-known cancer clinic, MD Anderson in Texas, was experimenting with this alongside its other treatments to help cancer patients. To explain this in its simplest form, since both foods are rich in Omega-3 fatty acids, they could decrease chemicals in the body related to cancer growth.

Since reading that MD Anderson was experimenting with it, even though they made it clear there was no evidence it could help patients with cancer, I was game. I ate the third cup of each, or something of the like, and nearly gagged for the next six hours. Since intermittent fasting was also something mentioned in the cancer-curing world, I figured at least I was fasting for a while, whether I liked it or not. After trying this only one more time, I was so nauseated I figured if I was meant to heal naturally, it would not include cottage cheese or flaxseed oil. Months later, I learned that I had a sensitivity to flaxseed oil—a near allergy to it—thus the natural and reflexive abhorrence for this terrible-tasting concoction. Sadly, I informed Russell that I had given his concoction a whirl, but my body couldn't tolerate it. He understood and agreed to stand with me in prayer for my healing.

Next, I heard from a woman who was recommended to me by a friend at church that the use of a castor-oil pack placed on the area with cancer could possibly help. Videos proclaimed great ease in the use of these packs and demonstrated ways to contain the oil successfully, even when used on the breast. Although doubtful of how oil would not defy gravity, I was still willing to try anything. My husband even entertained it and did not do any "boob-shaming" while I employed this technique. After applying the castor oil to my breast, I wrapped it in the gelatinous pack that was supposed to contain the oil. In case it didn't—and I was convinced it wouldn't—I wrapped that in plastic wrap and wore a sports bra and tank top that I didn't care about ruining in case the oil spilled out, and sat sedentary so as not to jostle and jiggle the oil unnecessarily. This attempt was a complete flop, and the oil drizzled and oozed through the pack and the plastic wrap, through the sports bra and out onto the tank top, and began to drip onto my stomach. If this technique were to work, I would have to be lying down, and that was not going to happen with loads of housework and more chapters to read in my cancer-curing quest. Determined not to waste the can of castor oil I ordered, I sequestered myself to the couch where I would sit like a potato after my mom or Tim had assisted me in the plastic wrap and straightjacket approach with the sports bra and the like. At the end of this clown show, I was determined to do only one thing—burn the sports bra and tank top that were supposed to be castor-oil-free in a bonfire in my yard. Since they were laden with copious amounts of oil, there was certain to be a full-blown, blazing fire!

Then there's the tale of the teas. Once, when driving back from San Diego, Julie implored me to take an alternate route through Phoenix to pick up a friend, only to drop him off in Bayfield so he could catch a ride from a stranger back to Pagosa, since she knew this was too much to ask of me after a thirteen-hour drive. To say he was talkative would be an understatement. My ninety-two-year-old dad used to say people like this were "vaccinated with a Victrola needle." Not only did he talk more than I did—and I can talk a blue streak—but he talked at such a rapid rate, with such intensity that my head was ready to explode before we got to the Sedona exit, and we still had six or seven hours to go. My gut impression was that he had done a little too much crystal meth or crack in his young life, but since we were stuck in the car for hours to come, no matter which way we sliced it, I shared with him that I was battling cancer. When I said, "I am trying to fight it naturally," he just about shouted at me. "Are you TRYING or are you DOING?!" Taken aback to say the least, and actually a bit offended, but perhaps equally convicted, I responded that I was trying everything I knew. He then dove into a diatribe about Yew tea, specifically a tea made from the bark of the Pacific Yew tree, and was prepared to be irritated if I hadn't tried it. Sheepishly, I let him know that not only had I not tried it but had never heard of it. He promised to send me some in exchange for the ride, and I assured him I would drink it. He also asked if I was taking CBD with THC, and when I stated I wasn't, he was indignant, coming close to scolding me for not looking into this. He said, "If you have cancer, and you are trying to cure it naturally, I am sure you have heard of this!" I assured him I had. This recurring theme about CBD with THC was beginning to ring in my ears.

His Pacific Yew tea—derived from the bark of the tree—arrived as he promised, and I begrudgingly drank it every day, but the taste was absolutely dreadful to me. With that bitterly bad taste, I figured it had to be doing something good. To keep in theme with the teas, my mom's friend, Carol Groseth, swore by the use of Essiac tea for cancer, since a relative had benefited from drinking it. Not accustomed to trying things suggested blindly, I researched this also, and found that it was named after a Canadian nurse named Rene Caisse (who named the herb after the reversal of her name). Made from a combination of burdock and rhubarb root, slippery elm, and sheep sorrel, it was linked to some remarkable medical success stories from those who'd used it. After ordering some, I realized making it was an arduous process. I needed to strain the herb, then steep it and cool it for twelve hours before drinking. It was such a large amount that I couldn't store it in my refrigerator, so I kept it cool outside on my porch at night. I only hoped the bears in my area didn't get curious. It, too, had a terrible taste, and I sipped it mostly, but ended up pinching my nose and simply gulping it down. The research didn't say that swallowing it or the Pacific Yew tea made it any less effective, so this is how I managed them. At least it didn't make me tremendously nauseated for hours on end like the cottage cheese and flaxseed combination!

Already giving Essiac tea a try, I resorted to another tea used in Mexico and given to me as a healing gift from a patient's daughter. This tea was homemade using guanabana leaves—thirteen to be exact, along with hot water to make this bland-tasting tea. How I came about this gift is somewhat peculiar. Being an overachiever by nature, I agreed to assist a very large and sedentary man named Forrest in and then out of an SUV so that he could enjoy an outing with his daughter. A fellow coworker, Michael Roman, also a therapist, was going to assist me in this arduous and overzealous endeavor. We would call this transfer a "dead lift." Perched between the car door and the patient's legs, sitting to make a transfer into a wheelchair placed next to the car, I reached around his hips for the waistband of his pants, said an internal "heave ho," and used momentum to lift him out of the car, Michael assisting from behind to lower him safely and securely into the wheelchair. Unaware that this elderly man had a guilty pleasure of Cheetos—which were sprinkled all over his shirt and pants and covering his fragile fingers—Michael and I successfully vaulted him into the WC only to discover that I was lathered with orange Cheeto dust on the front and back of my light grey shirt, and around the back of my khaki work pants, and even had a smear on the side of my cheek.

Feeling terrible that my work attire was bathed in a layer of this neon-colored cheesy film, his daughter said, "Oh, I am so sorry; is there anything I could get for you to make up for this and for helping my dad get out of the car?" She was well-known to me and knew from my frequent sessions with her father that I was battling cancer. Not able to receive gifts from patients of any significant amount, she thought to herself and then said, "Oh, I know of a tea that I can get for you that may help with your cancer. I will bring it to you the next time I see you." So that is the saga of how I ended up having leaves from the guanabana tree in Mexico. It was a mild and almost tasteless tea that I used for months, which may not have changed the status of my cancer, but warmed my throat and my spirit as well. Michael and I would break out into bouts of laughter about this colorful scene while finishing paperwork in our gym. And I believe I had to toss that grey T-shirt covered in Cheeto dust into the trash, as even "Shout-it Out" was not successful in removing the stains. It might as well have gone into the bonfire with the sports bra and tank top smeared in castor oil!

The last strange thing I tried was cold, kosher sauerkraut right out of the glass jar. This was recommended to me by a man whom I met along the way, who said he had cured his cancer naturally. A bit overzealous, I bought the largest jar I could find of kosher sauerkraut, but this had a similar effect as the cottage cheese mixture, and I was only able to manage that single jar of German kraut. Despite good intentions, I figured if I was going to heal, it was going to have to be without these cottage cheese and kraut potions. One may think I had lost it mentally, and after trying these odd methods, at times I felt like I was cursed, but when diagnosed with cancer, trust me, extreme measures are harnessed by many to try and cure it.

37

To Be or Not to Be

Sand was swiftly falling through the hourglass of my personal time-line when a decision would need to be made about whether or not I could avoid surgery. I took one more trip to Denver in October, and my fingers were crossed that the tumor had shrunk. All of my tried and true friends met with me as in the past, and I had warm welcomes in their homes and wonderful talks as always. Despite my earnest prayers, where I found myself up for hours at night asking God for healing, the dreaded phone call again came through as I reached the valley of brown farmlands on a rainy day. Since the nurse practitioner was calling me the very next day after the MRI, I knew I would not be hearing good news. With an alarmist tone, she said, "Kristi, the tumor has increased in size to 1.6 centimeters, and we have detected a second tumor that is almost 1 centimeter, and a possible third tumor that is 0.5 centimeters. I suggest you call the surgeon right away to take action." I thanked her for her prompt call and told her I would follow through. I wept as dark clouds enveloped me ascending Wolf Creek Pass, while a song from Tenth Avenue North called "Worn" sang about all that was dead inside being reborn. Feeling obviously worn, I wondered whether my healing journey was still a rational and realistic hope.

Having an already scheduled appointment with naturopath Dr. Stacy Mulkey to discuss the findings of this last test, I met her with tears streaming down my cheeks, telling her of the ever-growing and multiplying tumors. We both agreed it would be a waste to biopsy them, as we knew that at least one was definitely cancerous and that my only option at this time would be a mastectomy. She gave me the name of a female surgeon in Durango, who she commented was not a breast specialist, and suggested I call her as soon as possible. She comforted me by saying she knew I had tried everything I knew possible, and that I had followed all of her suggestions to the fullest. After giving her a hug and getting to my car, I googled the surgeon, found her number, and called without hesitation. I explained my plight to the receptionist, she asked for my MRI information, and I replied that I would send it.

Since the doctor's office was not allowed to receive the information I had requested without the MRI center sending it to me first, I finally—after multiple calls to the MRI center—was able to get my records emailed to the surgeon's office. After waiting to hear from them for a week, I called back and left another message that I had possibly three cancerous tumors and needed immediate attention to address this. I was frustrated, to say the least.

During this waiting period, I decided to casually "interview" some people I knew who'd had mastectomies as to what I could anticipate. Remembering that the wife of my dentist from San Diego almost died after she developed sepsis following her mastectomy and required six weeks or more of IV antibiotics in the hospital, I had a feeling of caution. One coworker from one of the rehab centers where I worked had a recent mastectomy, and I asked which surgeon she used, but unfortunately, he was no longer doing surgeries in this area. Then, I asked her how she felt about the process, and she responded matter-of factly, "I told the surgeon at my follow-up when he asked how I thought it went: Now I have one breast that is a stiletto and one that is an Ugg," meaning her original breast was rather attractive like a set of stiletto high heels, and the new breast was clunky like an Ugg boot or slipper. I had to restrain myself from laughing or crying. A few days after this, I asked another employee at another facility where I worked how her mastectomy went. She answered, "Well, I had some complications. After I had the spacers in for a while to heal my skin and was ready for my reconstruction, the surgeon asked me, "Do you want mom boobs or porn boobs?" I replied, "Just give me mom boobs." To this, I was already aghast at his terribly crude reference, which I felt was completely inappropriate. She then told me, "I developed an issue that is not so uncommon with that surgery. The new "mom boob" developed a calcification and was extremely hard and painful, so I had to have that removed and wait a while with the spacers again." For those of you unfamiliar with this, often after a mastectomy, weeks if not months go by while the skin is healing with "spacers" placed to separate the skin so the new breast can be inserted. She then proceeded to say, "When I went back to the surgeon, I told him, 'This time, give me porn boobs.'" I asked her sheepishly how long this process involving four surgeries took her, and she said, "It was just a few months shy of two years." My spirits were beginning to sink, and I hadn't even met with the local general surgeon, who wasn't even a breast specialist. After this, I was talking with a friend and her boyfriend, visiting from San Diego, about the fact that I was considering a mastectomy, and he said, "My ex-wife had cancer in one breast and, deciding to have both breasts removed, ended up having complications from both, leading to seven total surgeries." Truly, any comfort I thought I would receive from these casual interviews came crashing down on me, and feelings of dread swept over me. Although I was aware that mastectomies have saved the lives of many women with aggressive breast cancer, who had the genetic propensity for them to spread and recur, my heart was not in it. Since I had a non-aggressive, slow-growing type and had heard testimonies of people with my type healing without surgery or after a lumpectomy, I earnestly prayed that either my surgery would go flawlessly or I would be redirected in some way.

After waiting another week, I received no return phone call, so I brought my MRI records to the office and asked the administrative assistant if I could book an appointment. She commented that they had to review my records to ensure the need for surgery and then would return my call. Typically, surgeons are at the ready to book an appointment, so I was taken aback at their lackadaisical attitude toward addressing my cancer and proceeding with a surgical date. After waiting another week without a return call from their office, a new thought came to me. This feels in my soul like a message that this isn't the right time or surgeon to address this—if, after three attempts to get an appointment, they didn't have the decency to even call or email me with a message. Realizing they might be backlogged from the COVID-19 virus when they weren't allowed to address "non-emergent" cancer surgeries, I thanked God for the possible blessing this delay might bring to me, and I hoped that perhaps this surgery was not to be.

38

⚜

Turn in the Road

Dr. Mulkey recommended I get a thermography, a non-specific test that detects heat patterns in the body and could give me insight into my cancer. Working on a Saturday on my son's birthday, December 2, and having my medical records ready for my appointment later that day at five, Julie called and said, "Kristi, I wasn't able to print my medical forms at the library for my thermography, which is right before yours. Perhaps we can switch appointments, and if you can print off the forms at work and bring them to me, I can fill them out while you take my appointment." I told her this was no problem but ran into technical difficulties as the pages were printing with half of the information truncated and missing from the form. Noticing there was another employee named Amber working that day, younger and most likely more tech-savvy than me, I asked her for help. Amber ran over to the office where I was and said, "I don't mean to be nosy, but what's a thermography?" First, I told her I was battling cancer and went on to explain that it was a non-invasive way to monitor the breasts, avoiding a mammogram. It was not as specific but could reveal patterns, without smashing the already-existing tumor. She was intrigued and then said, "I am so sorry to hear you have cancer. What approach are you taking to battle it?" After telling her I was taking an alternative approach through a naturopathic doctor but was hitting roadblocks, I then said, "I have turned over every stone, but there is one missing link. My husband bought a few books for me on battling cancer, and in one book, titled *I Cure Cancer*, almost every doctor mentioned the use of Rick Simpson's Oil.[17] I said, "This oil is the only thing I haven't tried for my cancer, and I want to get it." She asked what it was. Feeling she was pressed for time, I quickly mentioned that it was an oil with CBD and THC meant to fight cancer. She had a quizzical look on her face and said, "CBD and THC?! Do you know if it has CBN in it?" I responded that I didn't know about CBN, and then she ran to the other side of the gym where she had been documenting and, like an inspired scientist, began typing and Google-searching. I didn't know what she was doing, but since she had corrected the computer error that was misprinting Julie's medical forms, I completed my printing task. She said, "Kristi, I had no idea about this oil and its benefits for cancer, but I just inherited a marijuana dispensary, and I believe I could get this oil for you!" I was dumbfounded. Already having stopped at a local dispensary—something totally uncharacteristic for me as I had never tried any type of drug OR been drunk—I was told they couldn't provide me with Rick Simpson's Oil, but they also informed me a small vial or month's supply would cost roughly $1,500. Telling Amber this story and that I would pay her whatever it was worth, I had to run to my thermography appointment and left her my number. As she was rushing to make a flight to Florida, I told her to have a wonderful time and figured I would talk to her when she returned.

To my surprise, while I was on Highway 3 that wound along the Animas River, with the sun beginning to set, I received an unexpected phone call from Amber. She said, "Kristi, do you have a minute before your

---

[17] Jacklin, *I Cure Cancer*, Chapters 1–6.

appointment?" I affirmed that I did, and she said, "I called my business partner and told him about your cancer battle and your need for Rick Simpson's Oil. He asked me, 'So your coworker, who is also a therapist and works with you helping the elderly, needs an oil that we can make, and will pay us whatever it costs?' Then he repeated the question, confirming that you are a therapist, same as me, and he replied, 'We will make this oil for her and give it to her as she helps others, and is a coworker and friend of yours. We won't take a dime from her.'" About to careen off the road over the guard rail and into the river, I regained my composure and, with tears streaming down my face, I said, "Amber, this gives me new hope! I feel I am being guided that I will heal this way and can avoid surgery." She was similarly overwhelmed and said she was behind me in this battle. Being that Amber, a therapist I had only met once before, had been there on a day I rarely worked, to fix the printer so I could print Julie's thermography paperwork that she randomly requested, that led to a conversation about a healing oil, I KNEW the stars were aligning and God was guiding me on this strange and winding road!

The thermography was helpful, and the nurse practitioner who specializes in oncology told me she was not alarmed by the MRI findings and for me to keep the faith and my instincts in tune. Since Julie was there waiting to have the next appointment, I was briefly able to share my good news with her about having access to Rick Simpson's Oil, and she was likewise excited about this unexpected gift from Amber and her work partner. I also shared the information with my mom and we were both astounded, stating, "What are the chances that you would both work on that Saturday when you both don't normally work, that you would share this information about your cancer battle that you hadn't even shared with more well-known to you therapists, and that you would come to the conclusion and mention you needed this marijuana oil, and she would say, 'Oh, I just inherited a marijuana dispensary and can make this priceless and expensive oil for you for free, as a gift?'" It was even Lukas's birthday—I couldn't make this stuff up! This was really happening, and a wave of hope swept over me. It just seemed too good to be true! In that moment, I was so thankful the surgeon's office hadn't taken the time to return my phone call. For now, the mastectomy was not to be.

39

The Power in a Green Leaf

Since my original diagnosis of stage zero cancer, my curious mind had been fascinated with the medicinal properties of marijuana for a few years now, and I had a familial link to this, too. My sister-in-law Debi Thomas's son, Micah, just so happened to be one of the largest CBD oil producers in California, and had been at the beginning of this wave that was crossing America. When Debi asked me if I would like to try the CBD oil to help fight my cancer, I was slightly hesitant. I really didn't know much about it, and with my upbringing and my position against all recreational drugs, I wasn't sure I could trust that this oil was untainted, and worried it might make me "high."

To match my inquisitive nature, I delved hard-core into the research behind it and discovered the mystery of the healing nature of the marijuana plant. One could say I was obsessed with a man named Dr. Mechoulam and his findings. I learned that Raphael Mechoulam was an Israeli-born biochemist and known as the Father of Cannabis, as he discovered the structure of cannabidiol (CBD) and delta 9-tetrahydrocannabinol (THC) in the 1960s, now used in the medical realm worldwide.[18] He went on to win six awards for his research, including the NIDA Discovery Award, and was the first to find that our brains, breasts, and bones had an endocannabinoid system that understood cannabis, unlike the pharmaceuticals so often prescribed. Since my early research, it has now been found that every organ of our bodies has an endocannabinoid system that understands the methods it employs. It has since been used to treat chronic pain, anxiety, depression and insomnia, glaucoma, MS, Alzheimer's, and ALS, to name a few, and some researchers are seeing anecdotal benefits for diseases like cancer. Arguably, the most astounding benefits are for children with epilepsy, as it has now been proven to decrease the amount of seizures in this patient population, which could change the brain and the lives of those who suffer from it.[19] Dr. Mechoulam studied cannabis for about sixty years, and since he was mostly interested in it for its chemical structure, after I was convinced of its amazing properties, I figured I should open my mind to its benefits. I insisted that my dad watch some of the videos, along with my mom, since he had taught high school health and had been on a staunch anti-drug and anti-marijuana campaign for decades. Discussions about pain would come up with my elderly patients nearly every therapy session, and although I wanted to tread lightly, I figured if I mentioned they look into it for treatment of their pain, this couldn't hurt. Two of my patients did full-blown research and actually called a doctor in LA who could measure and prescribe it, and they both had remarkable results with major pain relief.

---

[18] Jose Alexandre S. Crippa, et al, "Dr. Raphael Mechoulam, Cannabis and Cannabinoids Research Pioneer (November 5, 1930–March 9, 2023) and His Legacy for Brazilian Pharmacology," *Brazilian Journal of Psychiatry* 45, no. 3 (2023): 201–202, doi: 10.47626/1516-4446-2023-0047.

[19] Richard J. Huntsman, "Cannabis for Pediatric Epilepsy," *Journal of Clinical Neurophysiology* 37, no. 1 (2020): 2–8, https://pubmed.ncbi.nlm.nih.gov/31895184/.

My nephew gave me some CBD to try for insomnia, which I've battled since I came out of the womb, and although it didn't have any marked effect, I wondered if it could help fight my cancer, so I used it for this as well. I learned upon further reading in the book *I Cure Cancer* that to battle cancer, THC was an important component. I would need to bite the bullet and go against my lifelong drug-free stance and try this green plant that many enjoyed and others warned as a gateway drug to more dangerous drugs.

Just about the time I was convinced to try this wonder drug, we had visitors I'd known my entire life stop at our house for a few hours on their way from Colorado Springs to San Diego. Leigh and Eric Grinstaff had moved to Colorado Springs just after I moved to Denver, and since I knew Leigh and had vacationed with her family since I was a baby, I was comfortable discussing my health issues with her. After informing her that my cancer was not improving, but was slowly growing and multiplying, Eric, who was casually lounging on the couch but not engaging in our conversational catch-up until that time, blurted out, "Have you ever heard of that RSO?" I asked what RSO was, and he replied, "Rick Simpson's Oil." Aha, I should have known. Then he said, "I had a friend who had a golfball-sized cancerous tumor on his neck, and he took that RSO, and his tumor disappeared." Leigh corroborated this story, and my jaw dropped—I was astounded! This Rick Simpson's Oil kept circling back in many conversations about my cancer. When I felt I could speak, I said to Eric, "I feel I'm going to recover from this cancer, and if I try this oil, and my cancer disappears like your friend's did, would you mind if I wrote about this moment in a book I might write?" He calmly and quietly welcomed the idea. Since I had tried everything else under the sun to fight my cancer, I decided to take a step off the ledge and try this green-leafed marvel.

40

Elmore's Corner

A friend at church knew I had sleep problems and also suggested a marijuana oil that had some THC in it that she said might help. She knew the importance of sleep for overall well-being and encouraged me to try it. She told me the woman who made it wanted to remain anonymous and agreed to meet somewhere neutral. We chose Elmore's Corner. Here I was in my fifties, never having been drunk or tried anything illegal in my life—even though it was legal in Colorado—and I would be doing a drug exchange at a local convenience store. It was almost unbelievable that I wasn't able to get this at the nearest dispensary or from a doctor who knew the exact dose I should take. My friend handed me the oil in a small glass bottle with a dropper and instructed me to take a few drops at bedtime. I must admit, since I had battled insomnia for so long, this oil did help me sleep for the short time I took it. Taking a drop or two every night, I knew I would run out eventually, but my friend said her connection couldn't guarantee she could make it exactly the same way every time. Again, being a science-minded person, I was frustrated that this wasn't something that could be prescribed to me.

A month or so after Amber surprised me with the offer to have her work partner make Rick Simpson's Oil for me, she called me and said, "I am so sorry it took me a while to get this oil to you." I assured her I was beyond grateful whenever she was ready with this amazing gift. She said, "I wish you could come to my dispensary to get it, but since I'll be handing it off to you, I have to ask you something unusual." I quickly responded, "Can you meet me at a random place like Elmore's Corner?" We both had to laugh. Here we were, both health care professionals, she with a doctorate, and again, I was lowered to a clandestine drug exchange in the parking lot of a local store. It felt so odd. When we first discovered that I needed it, and she owned the dispensary, we both looked for a clinical trial to see if there was any scientific credence in its use for breast cancer or any cancers. She found none. Mentioning that I wanted to be a part of a clinical trial, she agreed, but we had no way of performing our own. Even mentioning this to my friend Andrea Cordle's husband, who was an ER doctor, he was not sure how I would join a study. My mind knew I had to try it, but I did not want an excessive dose that would cause any psychedelic effects. Amber wished the same thing for me.

In the end, we did not choose Elmore's Corner for our exchange but another undisclosed parking lot. She was going to leave it on the front wheel of my car, but I felt leaving a sought-after product that was quite costly would be too risky, so we were able to meet face-to-face for the exchange. She had the oil in a syringe and said to take a very small amount of it. Thanking her perhaps too profusely, I gave her a hug and told her, "I believe you will be a pivotal part of my journey to recovery."

That night, I gently squeezed the syringe, and the oil did not budge. She told me it had a tarry quality, and it truly seemed harder than tree sap. I squeezed a little harder, and way too much erupted from the top of the syringe. Since this was like brown gold, I retracted the handle of the syringe, and to my great relief, the tarry oil made its way back into the syringe, and I was able to administer a tiny amount under my tongue. Unfortunately, it had a paradoxical effect on my sleep. Known to make the majority of its users fall swiftly and deeply to sleep, I was wired for sound like a chipmunk on crack. Talking about being wired, I also became extremely creative. One night after taking my ever-so-infinitesimal dose, I was wide-eyed with thoughts circling in my mind and whole paragraphs of eight different books with separate titles zipping around in my brain. One woman at church said I was spinning, while another at work said I was an Energizer Bunny.

Since some of those chapters are now a part of this book, I wondered if God really did have something up his sleeve when he created this mind-blowing green plant. After many nights with barely any sleep, a thought came to me that I needed to take it in the morning before work rather than at night, hoping its half-life would drain out of my body by nightfall. This did help for the first month, and my work productivity was off the charts, but my rate of speech was a bit rapid, and I had to employ some self-calming measures before entering a patient's room to make sure I didn't startle them like a bull in a china shop. Amber was able to give me one more month's supply during this attempt to improve naturally. With thoughts of future non-profit books swirling in my mind, I figured the RSO oil would be of benefit no matter what.

41

✦

A Time of Testing

March had arrived, and it was time to make my pilgrimage to Denver for the final test before I needed to make my decision about a surgical mastectomy. In my spirit, I felt I would heal naturally—I truly believe I had heard from God that surgery wouldn't be necessary. I again met with my wonderful friends, but two visits stood out to me. First, with Nicki Shier, with whom I started my young career at Mercy Hospital in Denver. We sat in her car and prayed, and she affirmed to me that she was supporting me and believed that with everything I was doing, I could heal.

Next, after perhaps twenty-two years, I reunited with a former house-mate of mine and his wife—he lived on the main level of the house and I rented the upstairs apartment. Years before, a successful businessman in his twenties and dating a woman who was, in my opinion, not the optimal girl for him, I urged him to end that relationship and consider dating some-one who would complement him. Since I worked in a rehab center with therapists, 99 percent of whom were women, I came across the classiest and most vibrant speech therapist, and thought the instant I met her, "She could be the woman for Jim." She must have thought I was crazy because I had only talked with her one time. The next time I did, I said, "Sherri,

I have this fabulous neighbor and friend named Jim Stirbis, and he is successful, kind, thoughtful, and just a great guy, and I was wondering if you would go on a blind date with him?" She looked a bit stunned, but agreed to give it a whirl. The minute I got home from work, I called Jim and said, "Hey, I met this fabulous girl at work, and I know you will think she is incredible and you will be attracted to her in many ways. I asked her if she would consider going on a date with you, and she said yes, so you have to give her a call." He, too, must have thought I was out of my mind to offer him up as a date without asking him first, but he said he would call. In my memory, he didn't call right away. I asked her at work if he'd called, and she said he hadn't yet, so again, that evening, I called him and asked if he was going to follow through with it. I told him, "If you don't, I know you will be missing out on someone wonderful." He called her, and they had a date at Red Rocks, and he called me the next day and said, "Kristi, I think I met the girl I will marry." To say that I was over the moon would be an understatement, and after he sent her flowers, she was smitten, and the rest is history. They had a December wedding and have been married for over twenty years! Although they met Lukas when I first adopted him, and I had been in Denver since that time, I hadn't been able to visit with them. This time, I gave Sherri a call, letting her know I would be in the area for a few days, and they offered to host me for a night before the ultrasound I had scheduled in Colorado Springs. We had a terrific time, catching up on our lives and our kids' lives, and also updating them on my health status. Knowing they were concerned about the cancerous tumors I had not yet had surgery on, they nonetheless said they were supporting me in my journey and were hoping for the best.

Next, I met with a friend named Jessica Yackley, whom I also knew as a coworker when I worked at Casa de las Campanas in San Diego. Jessica was a rehab aide in the therapy department, and a few decades younger than me. Being much more computer-savvy than me and most people in my generation, she was instrumental in helping me upload photos for my first book, "The Child Who Listens," about Lukas's adoption. Being an aide, her intention was to use it as a launchpad for a career as a therapist or chiropractor. Her choice to pursue a doctorate in chiropractic work was linked to its scope of practice, including a whole-body approach to healing. She asked me to be a reference for her when applying to a school in Iowa, and I was pleased to do so. While she was in chiropractic school, expanding her knowledge of the links between what we eat, drink, and do in life with cancer, she tried to help her mother overcome her battle with cancer, but unfortunately lost her to the dreadful disease. She told me over the phone, on one of my nature walks near my Durango home, that her focus as a chiropractor would include helping those who struggled with cancer.

She explained that her last internship before graduation would be in Denver, and we should attempt to get together. Excited to see her complete her three arduous years of school, I told her I would be having one more test on my cancer in the Springs, and she was grateful the timing would align with the final months of her internship. We couldn't have orchestrated this if we tried! There was a feeling of inspiration and hope I felt simply learning that we would meet and have the chance to exchange ideas about methods to improve my health.

When we sat down at a natural fast-food restaurant in Denver, called Modern Market Eatery, I began to tell her about my recent health updates, and she said, "Kristi, I feel the doctors are missing something." She repeated this and said, "Since I have been at chiropractic school, I have begun to understand more about how the body works as a whole. I have also discovered a faith in God and feel he has designed us to heal." She encouraged me to keep digging and to find the missing link in my health mystery. She said, "I really feel you may be able to avoid surgery, and I will be here as a sounding board if you have any questions. I really think they're missing something."

Knowing I had written one book and was in the process of writing my second, she also mentioned, "I also feel I am called to write a book, and it will be focused on God's design for our bodies to heal." Excited to hear about this, we explored this topic, and I encouraged her to write it when she had time after taking her board exams and beginning her career. Mentioning that I thought my friend and publisher would be interested in the book, I affirmed that she should get in touch with me when she was ready to publish her work, even if that was years away.

Returning to my friends' Karin and Djimmer's house, where I would spend my last night in Denver, before driving to the Springs for my next test, I felt divine peace with that sentence ringing in my ear, "Kristi, I believe they are missing something." A confidence flooded over me that I was soon to discover the missing puzzle piece in this now eight-year battle. It was as if the answer was just waiting to be discovered. I also heard a voice telling me that the test the next day may confirm the cancer was still there, but I wasn't to worry. Having time for a walk with Karin and her loyal and loving pitbull, Bambi, later that day, I shared my thoughts with her, and she repeated that she would support all of my decisions, but also told me to be wise and not to wait too long if surgery was needed. Assuring her I would heed her advice, I slept soundly in her home that night and prepared myself for the ultrasound, which would give me immediate feedback on my health status. All the while, the words spoken by Jessica stayed with me: "I believe they are missing something."

As I drove from Denver to Colorado Springs, snow falling on my windshield, I had a sense telling me the tumors were still there, but not to fear. Jessica and the time shared with her had prepared me for this, but inspired me and gave me hope that this would not necessarily mean I was at the end of the road. One more step felt like it was in my future. So I drove with a certain peace, despite the news I was feeling destined to hear. Arriving at the office, I was just recovering from a cold. With throat lozenges quelling my incessant cough and the scratchy sound of my voice, and a blue surgical mask covering my face, I was paranoid that if I sounded sick, they would turn me away due to COVID panic. A female technician whisked me back into a dark room and, after I changed into a gown, instructed me to lie on the treatment table. Since she was taking quite a while and circling around repeatedly, I instinctively knew there was a problem area she was focused on. Then the words I dreaded: "I have found some very dense tissue, but also areas of concern, and I need to call in the doctor who is more well-versed to further test you." Not my first rodeo, I knew this wasn't going to be good news. A male doctor walked into the room and, proceeding to repeat the tech's words, explained what I already felt in my heart and mind, that he was there since the ultrasound was more complicated than normal. After quite a while longer, he confirmed, "Kristi, we have found two tumors, and possibly a third." I mentioned to him that my recent MRI had shown the same results. With this added information, he spoke candidly, saying, "I'm sorry to have to tell you this, but you need to schedule an appointment with a surgeon for a mastectomy as soon as possible. There is a wonderful breast surgeon here in Colorado Springs that I can recommend. I wouldn't waste any time, and I have confidence in the surgeon and your prognosis if you have surgery to remove the cancer, since I don't believe it has advanced to your lymph."

Thanking him for his direct approach and concern, I extended my hand to thank him, and he assured me the front office would have the name and number of the breast surgeon. He wished me the best, and I again told him I appreciated his time and expertise, all the while holding back the tears welling up in my eyes, ready to spill unabashedly onto my cheeks.

Leaving the office with no one having noticed my cough or throat symptoms and placing me in quarantine, I made it to my car, and once on I-25 headed home, immediately calling my mom to tell her the terrible news. Reaching her at an inopportune time—or so I thought at that moment—when she was getting her haircut, I let her know I didn't mind if the stylist heard my travails. Weren't hair stylists like therapists anyway, hearing way more information than they bargained for when they signed up to "coif" someone's hair?

Before plunging straight in, I excitedly told her about my meeting with Jessica. Mentioning that this had lit a flame of hope in me, I told her I felt I was going to receive news that would give me direction, but I didn't know from where. Presuming I was on speaker phone with the stylist stranger, I gave my mom the diagnosis bomb that confirmed what they found on the ultrasound. None of the teas, or castor-oil wraps, or diets had worked thus far, and the two, possibly three, tumors were still there.

Surprisingly—but in a way, what I had been spiritually prepared for—my mom said, "Kristi, I was telling the hair stylist about your test today, and I told her that you had a feeling the tumors were still there, and she said to me, 'There is a doctor in Bayfield that has a different type of test. It looks at the whole body, and he was able to reverse his own cancer that was considered irreversible.' I really feel this is it! Just like Jessica said, I think they are missing something, and he is going to figure it out." Insane as all of this may sound, I couldn't help but agree. I felt this hope, this confidence that was not natural. It felt supernatural. Rather than allow fear to enter in, I drove with a peace that passed understanding. As I approached Wolf Creek Pass, where I had just been crying tears of despair after my MRI several months earlier, I cried tears of thankfulness for the healing that was possibly to come. As I drove along the road that mirrored the winding river cascading from the majestic mountains, and passed the pine trees that pointed toward the heavens, that peace settled into my soul. With terrible results just confirmed, I knew it was not natural for me to feel this way. Ascending that 10,000-foot mountain, rain splashed my windshield as a song by Blanca called "The Healing" came on the radio. It talked about God bringing healing to us, followed by Zach Williams' "Heaven Help Me" about someone calling to heaven for help and to believe in a time of desperation. I knew I was getting close to the end of the road—either my path would bring surgery or it would bring natural healing. I prayed this doctor would have time to see me quickly and that he would guide me in the direction I had searched for for years.

42

The Missing Link

Not wasting precious time after I arrived home, I called this practitioner named Dr. Chris Kaufmann that Wednesday, and he surprisingly returned my call the next day when I was home with time on my hands. Without hesitation, after hearing my diagnosis, he said, "No one knows I am back in town after taking time off, so I could see you tomorrow, on Friday, if you are free." Flabbergasted that I might be able to see him the following day, my hopes began to surge. Finding out that I had breast cancer, he delved into some health questions straight out of the gate. He first asked, "What is your body temperature?" I responded that I was frequently cold and had battled with a low body temperature of 96.5 for years. He responded, "That tells me your thyroid is struggling." Next, he asked, "Do you have irregular periods and are you still menstruating?" I mentioned that yes, at fifty-five, I was still menstruating and did have an irregular cycle, to which he commented about a hormonal imbalance. Lastly, he asked, "Have you ever had a root canal?" I answered that I had, many years ago, before my cancer began, and that I was having pain in that tooth and had been to a dentist to address it. To the dentist's defense, I skipped the X-rays he offered as I was paying out of pocket, and he covered an area of the tooth and said that if the pain persisted, he would need to do further testing and may have to perform a more extensive procedure. Dr. Chris then commented, "Dentists and some doctors are finding a link between root canals and breast cancer." Then, with a form of excitement, as if he were a detective, he said, "Humor me and look up a chart linking this tooth to areas of the body. Which tooth is it?" I told him, and he himself looked it up and, with a passion in his voice, exclaimed, "That tooth is linked to the mammary sinus. Please come tomorrow if you can, and let's see if we can figure out what is driving this cancer."

With a feeling of relief settling over me, I felt this could be the person who would unearth the mystery I had been trying to figure out for years. I went downstairs where my mom lived and retold her everything he said, and she started to cry and gave me a hug and said, "Kristi, I think this is it. I think he is going to discover what has been happening in your body. This doctor is going to help you heal from cancer!" Embracing her with tears streaming down my cheeks, I responded, "Mom, I think this may be the answer I have been looking for."

Driving to his house the next morning, the positive energy in me was palpable. A new hope had been birthed in me the day before. I could barely wait to get to his office! Traveling down a dirt road that took me over the Pine River on a one-lane wooden bridge, I thought to myself, *Finding him would be like finding a needle in a haystack. He is literally "over the river and through the woods," but lives in the same town as I do.* Arriving at his house a few minutes early, I knocked at the door—a golden retriever and a black labrador lounging beside it—and was greeted by a man with bright eyes and a vibrant smile—a stark contrast to some of the radiologists and one surgeon I'd met during this health crisis. He welcomed me into his home and explained that he would be testing me with a machine that measured frequencies, also used in Austrian emergency rooms for diagnostic purposes. He had a metal probe that pressed into pressure points in my hand and explained that an abnormal measurement below a fifty would signal sickness. When he measured my left and healthy breast, the measurement was a perfect fifty, and when he tested my right breast laden with cancer, the measurement was a ten. He explained this was a form of confirmation that the right breast was "unhealthy." Then, after placing my hand on a metal device and waiting for the machine to calibrate, he read the results that showed I had mammary carcinoma and also "odontoid sepsis," the latter of which I understood was a dental infection. He commented, "I'm also finding that you have an MSG sensitivity," to which I responded, "Wow! I never told you that, but MSG is thought to be the culprit that sent me into anaphylactic shock, and something that gave me severe headaches before that." He continued, "I have referred people to the dentist I'm recommending, and he has told me his X-rays have missed infections that my machine never has." He then directed me, saying, "Get to the dentist right away. Don't do anything else before you do that. I think you have a tooth infection from your root canal that has been festering unseen for years. Call him right away." He also gave me some topical iodine to rub on my breast until that time, explaining that an iodine deficiency also predisposed me to breast complications. He welcomed me to do contrast baths using his sauna and the river next to his home any time I wanted. He intuitively instructed me not to "overwork" and take time to calm my system to allow healing, all things I knew I needed to do.

Leaving his home and driving back over the wooden bridge, wondering just what led me to him and to his home in the middle of the woods and the middle of nowhere, I knew in my heart it was a God-send. In my spirit, I felt this was the missing piece of the puzzle I had been waiting to find. This may be what my friend Jessice was referring to when she said, "They are missing something, Kristi. I know they are missing something." Hope was the only feeling that remained.

43

The Root Cause

My friend Erica Viviani, a fellow physical therapist whom I met when I gave her a tour of Mercy Medical Center in Denver during her interview, was the first person who introduced me to functional medicine. This form of medicine hunts for the root cause of sickness and disease, looking at all systems of the body to unearth the cause of the body expressing itself in illness. She and her husband, Jerome Stewart, were instrumental in cheering me on and supporting me during this trying time in my life. As mentioned earlier, they had brought my attention to Dr. Stengler in Encinitas through a video they sent, also featuring Nasha Winters, who started Namaste, where I was currently receiving care for my cancer. My doctor, Dr. Stacy Mulkey, had already asked me whether or not I had mercury amalgams, to which I answered that they had already been removed, and thus she would have no idea that a root canal I had years prior could be linked to my cancer. After calling Erica to tell her that this "frequency machine" detected a tooth infection, she encouraged me to go right away, stating that this could be one of the reasons I was struggling with cancer.

Having to wait until Monday to call Dr. Rothchild, the dentist, since his office was closed on Friday when I got his number, I heard back from the receptionist saying she had a several-month wait for new patients. Fearing that I may have to wait for several months, I explained my plight and my several-year battle with breast cancer, and that Dr. Chris referred me because he detected an infection that might be driving my cancer. She said she would get back to me later that week, and, no sooner had I hung up than I received a return call from her that the doctor was concerned for my situation, and would "squeeze" me into the schedule that week. Little did I know, his office was literally a few hundred yards away from my workplace, and I could get away from work and fit it in on Wednesday, hours before a flight I had planned that same afternoon to go visit my family in Pittsburgh for a special event. Feeling things were aligning quickly as I needed them to, I affirmed I would absolutely be there for that appointment, and I thanked the receptionist, also named Kristi, for considering the gravity of my situation and fitting me into a busy schedule. She answered that the doctor insisted after hearing I had cancer and didn't have time to waste.

Remembering that day vividly, I found myself standing in a high-tech, dome-like structure with an instrument that made a sweeping movement and, wondering what it might find, I prayed the doctor would find something wrong with my tooth. Never before would I wish this for myself, but I wanted to think there was hope for recovery. Feeling I had exhausted every other avenue, this was my last effort.

After the X-ray and sitting in the comfortable, reclining dental chair, with purplish hues cast on the painted walls and artwork that featured blooming flowers-a stark contrast to some of the bare, dismal offices I had been to along the way—a feeling of anticipation and calm settled over me. Dr. Rothchild entered the room with a seasoned aura and a similar enthusiasm to Dr. Chris's, and he exclaimed, "Kristi, I heard Dr. Chris referred you to me. Well, he was right again! Not only is your tooth infected, but the jaw is infected on the same side for several inches. It's the same tooth where you had your root canal." Almost unbelievably similar to Dr. Chris, he said, "Let's look at the chart linking the tooth to areas of the body." Then, after pursuing the chart, he said, "Oh, yes, that tooth is linked to the mammary sinus. I believe the toxins from the tooth could have drained into your breast." He then asked, "Have you had any issues with your left breast?" I told him the left breast hadn't had any issues or calcifications that were indicative of possible cancers. I also mentioned I had tried every diet under the sun to try to reduce or rid myself of the cancer. Then, with confidence and a warm expression on his face, he said, "Kristi, let's get this tooth extracted, and then return to the diet you mentioned, and hope that your cancer goes away." Anecdotally mentioning a link between root canals and breast cancer, he mentioned that he wished me the best and wanted me to keep him updated on my progress.

Leaving his office and heading straight to the airport to fly to Pittsburgh, I couldn't wait to meet with my parents, who would join me on that flight and tell them the news. Once we all made it through security, I was able to share everything Dr. Rothchild told me. As the flight lifted off the ground, my spirits soared in equal time. The looming threat of cancer further invading my body for years to come, and an upcoming mastectomy seemed to fade away. Was it ironic that an infected dental root may just be the root cause of my disease? I was soon to find out.

44

❖

Honoring My Father

M y mom, dad, and I made it smoothly to Pittsburgh and were hosted by my cousin Lesley Mueller, who made special efforts to make this trip a memorable one. This trip would include two celebrations, one for her father and one for mine. Her dad would celebrate his ninetieth birthday, and mine would enjoy a celebration of a basketball achievement.

Lesley had been one of my dad's biggest basketball fans from afar, living with us one summer and attending every summer league game, becoming familiar and friends with all the players, and having a crush on one of them, named Matt. She even traveled hours to witness my dad's Abington High School team win the Pennsylvania State Division 1 Championship. After spending this spring day walking the beautiful cherry blossom tree-lined streets with Lesley's daughter, Joan, and her precious pup, Bennie, I remembered why I enjoyed the East Coast so much. That feeling of moisture in the air, the sweet aromas, and the lush green and pink tulips and yellowish daffodils that sprinkled the hillsides and the neighbors' yards. Every ounce of my body with all its senses soaked in every ounce that it had to offer.

The first day, my mom, dad, Lesley, and Joan met my cousin Sara at my Uncle Charlie's nursing home to celebrate his birthday, with a wonderful cake to top it off. Some of the residents even poked their heads in the room that was reserved for the special time, saying that Charlie was a delightful man to be around, and also could be counted on for any updates or stats on the Pittsburgh Pirates, of which he was one of the most avid and longtime fans. At this late stage in his life, he would call not only my dad but also his daughter, Becky, to review game plays, hits, and wins or losses. Perhaps this sports madness ran in our family, something in our blood and our bodies, a gift we were grateful for.

After spending time visiting Uncle Charlie and enjoying time spent with family, it was time for the next event. Lesley, Joan, and I picked up Julie at the airport in Pittsburgh, and we drove on a calm, rainy day through the winding roads of Pennsylvania to our destination. My dad would be receiving an honor at his alma mater, West Virginia Wesleyan, in the town of Buckhannon, also where my mom was born and had attended college. When my dad, Jim (a.k.a. Wilkie), went to Wesleyan, he was the co-captain of the baseball and basketball teams. His co-captain for both teams, Gary Hess—who he had known for upwards of seventy years—was also making the drive out for this celebration with his wife, Carolyn, and their daughter, Laurie. My mom was a cheerleader for the basketball team, and while she was out on the court with her dapper outfit gathering enthusiasm for the team, he noticed her as a freshman, and the rest is history. Gary, along with every other teammate except for my dad, had already been inducted into the college's Hall of Fame.

When it came time for my dad to receive the honor, he joked that he was glad they allowed him to receive it before he was dead and buried, being that he was almost 90 years old. He gave thanks to his teammates, without whom he wouldn't have been able to achieve this honor. His team during his senior year made it to the elite eight in the country, and although they lost by a few points, the opposing team had players who made it into the NBA. To this day, this team made it the farthest in the March

Madness Tournament. They made it to the Sweet Sixteen during his junior year, and due to this success, the entire squad would finally be in the Hall of Fame. It was a wonderful time for him to be recognized for a game he was passionate about and was still dedicated to at this age. Actually, he was still coaching at the local college, Fort Lewis in Durango, and he assisted the coach in leading the team to the playoffs just a few weeks prior. He has been coaching since he graduated from college in 1959, and for this, I was so proud. A part of me hoped that the pendulum would swing in my favor to round out the remaining months of this year with good news.

45

The Welcomed Extraction

That providential day in May arrived for my tooth extraction, and I recall sitting in the dental chair telling Dr. Rothchild that I was most likely the most eager and excited person ever to receive a dental extraction in his or any dentist's career. Deep down, I felt certain this was one of the main reasons I had developed breast cancer. Knowing that many factors contributed to it, including my compromised immune system, and perhaps environmental factors to say the least, I felt this tooth and jaw infection, and the subsequent inflammation that leached into my glands on a daily basis, was hopefully linked to my breast cancer, as some had surmised. This was truly my last hope. Dr. Rothchild chuckled, saying no one in his forty-plus-year career had ever uttered the words that they were looking forward to having their tooth pulled.

Thinking back, my root canal procedure had been several years before my first diagnosis of stage zero breast cancer, and isolated to my right side, so this theory could hold ground. As motivated as I was to hit the ground running with my diet right after the surgery, the simple fact was that initially, I could only eat soft foods like yogurt and ice cream that were most likely not going to be a part of my healing plan.

The extraction involved more pressure on my jaw than I imagined, and he did a cavitation procedure on my jaw, which he explained included micro drilling into the bone that would get rid of the sepsis and allow the bone to regrow and heal without residual infection. He told me I could take arnica for pain, but I must admit, this was not enough to quell the gnawing ache in my jaw, and I had to rely on acetaminophen for a few days to remain comfortable.

During my recovery, Tim ordered a few more books I'd requested, one titled *How to Starve Cancer Without Starving Yourself* by Jane McLelland. She, like me, was a physical therapist with a science-based mind and a mostly healthy lifestyle, and she, like me, also had a sweet tooth. Maybe that tooth had been trying to tell me something for years. My predilection for it may have also been my nemesis. Her research went far beyond mine, and she stated in one chapter that some oncologists even had to study her work and findings to become better oncologists. I was not at this level in biochemistry at all, but I admired her tenacity, and while reading it thought, "If she could beat the odds and the death sentence the oncologists had given her, I can overcome it too."

As I recall, she had ovarian cancer, which later spread to her lungs, and she was given months, possibly only weeks, to live. She unearthed science that had been discovered decades prior, and since she found out that cancer fed on sugar, she had a genius idea. She was attempting to stop the cancer from growing, not believing she could heal, but hoping for a few more years as a newly married woman. This idea was to ask her doctor if she could take Metformin, typically used for diabetics, to control blood sugar. She deduced that if Metformin was used to control blood sugar, perhaps it could help her body control the sugars in her body and slow the cancer growth.[20] This brought to mind an idea Erica's husband,

---

[20] Jane McLelland, *How to Starve Cancer Without Starving Yourself: One Woman's Extraordinary True Story of Courage, Survival, and a Discovery That Could Transform the Lives of Millions* (Agenor Publishing, 2018), 107.

Jerome, had given me. He told me to try taking Berberine, which was a natural sugar controller. Since I didn't think I could get a doctor to give me Metformin, when I was ready to go "all in," I would try Berberine as a substitute for Metformin. It may not work, but I figured it couldn't hurt. Jane came up with a protocol that researchers at renowned oncology centers are now using as a guide. Being a biology major, I had a hard time digesting everything she included in this protocol but gleaned the pertinent information related to me, and readied myself to avoid refined sugar or alcohol as I "starved" the cancer.

Another gem I learned from Jerome was that broccoli sprouts contain the chemical sulforaphane, which may have a preventive agent for cancer, since he explained it was anti-inflammatory and caused apoptosis or cell death in cancer cells. This would also be in my arsenal of supplements, but I wanted to do some final testing to ensure my body could accommodate these supplements. Now that my toxic tooth was history, I felt momentum to take the final steps toward healing.

To add to my momentum, one day while outside on a walk, a text message pinged my phone, and I noticed it was from my friend and former coworker, Tanya Becker. She was with me at work in the rehab gym at Casa de las Campanas when I received the phone call with my original diagnosis. Also being a science-minded woman due to her own autoimmune issues, she'd sent me the number for Mario, who had reversed stage IV cancer that had spread from his prostate to his liver and elsewhere, and meeting with him was a major catalyst in my quest for natural healing. I noticed she'd sent me a new video about a cancer survivor. Today, it's curiously been removed from the internet, but he also wrote a book about his experience healing from colon cancer.

Since it was a warm, late spring day, I decided to listen to his video interview while sitting on a bench I referred to as my prayer bench that overlooked the powerful San Juan Mountains. I asked for guidance while listening to it, and knew it would be inspiring. Not able to find or recall his name, my hope is that you'll trust this information is true. Since I listened intently to every word, I recall many details, including that he was from France and owned about twenty Jiu-Jitsu gyms in New York City. Shockingly, since he was a very healthy man who prided himself on his personal fitness, which included a non-processed food diet, he was diagnosed with colon cancer. He had a male relative who also had colon cancer, but he attributed this to the relative's unhealthy lifestyle. After his diagnosis, one factor stuck out to him like a sore thumb—stress. Knowing that this was now a proven link to many cancers, he realized that during COVID, these multiple gyms, which were his main livelihood, were closed down, making no money, and he was spiraling downward financially into a crisis situation. He deduced that this could likely be the main reason he developed cancer, that, and a possible genetic propensity toward its expression. Discovering, like many of us who want to heal naturally, that cancer feeds on sugar, he decided he needed to be even more strict with his diet, and, reading up on fasting, he would incorporate this into his regimen. He would have opted out of chemo, but his six-centimeter tumor was restricting bowel movements, so he had no choice but to try it. He decided on three rounds of chemo to shrink the tumor, and hoped to avoid it after this. He recalled that while sitting in the chair receiving chemo, he was frequently offered treats containing sugar. Although he wanted to scream at the top of his lungs to everyone sitting there that they were feasting on the very thing the chemo was trying to kill, he politely declined the nurse's offer, stating it was not part of his regimen. While strictly fasting from all foods during chemo, he interestingly had absolutely no side effects from the powerful chemical therapy. He incorporated five- to seven-day fasts, something that didn't particularly resonate with me, but I was amazed at his tenacity in being able to do this.

As for his diet, he ate red organic beef, mostly steak, only green vegetables, and no fruit or sugar of any type, to achieve an alkaline pH. "Greens" resonated with me as I love all vegetables save for lima beans and peas, possibly due to their gritty, mushy texture. He deviated from his strict diet only once, when his mother, a pastry chef from France, came to visit him for the Christmas holiday. He admitted that he craved her baking treats, especially during the festive season, and indulged in his mother's home-made croissants and pastries on a daily basis for a week—and he savored every bite. After this unapologetic and gluttonous week of luscious baked goods, he returned to fasting and his beef and greens diet. To his oncologist's amazement, the large tumor had all but disappeared in four months with the three rounds of chemo combined with his diet and fasting technique. As I sat on my prayer bench, getting ready for my own protocol to begin, I was inspired by this man's story and thankful for Tanya investing time in my healing and sending this video. Just what would my healing entail, I was not sure. But I prayed I would know in time.

46

The Rainbow Connection

The night was vivid in my memory, and trying to avoid waking Tim, I went to a set of steps near our garage and called my friend Lana to ask her for guidance and prayer. I had heard of so many diets, and had tried a vegan diet, but my body just didn't feel well with this. While talking to her, I remember saying, "I wish God would just tell me what to eat!!" She asked a few questions while we talked, and I recall telling her that our well water couldn't be used because the pump had broken, and she said with intensity, "The well water! I feel there is a reason it is broken. You are not supposed to drink that water the way it is!" She felt this idea had been divinely sent, and with the Camp Lejeune commercials about the link between contaminated water and cancer, I knew why. With compassion, she asked me additional questions about others I had talked to who had healed naturally. Telling her one story of the woman named Chris who ate a vegan diet, she said emphatically, "Where was that woman when she healed?" I stated she was in Costa Rica. Lana said with conviction, "She was by the ocean, and where are we? We live near cows, salmon in streams, and have organic farmers with organic beef. I feel God is letting you know you can eat local meat and things that are grown here." Her message was clear, simple, and succinct, and I resonated with it. My excitement continued to mount.

Since it was nearing midnight, I crept quietly into my bedroom to charge my phone since my battery was running low. My charger was next to a window that overlooked my backyard, which was so very dry. I had been praying for rain, but the ten-day forecast had none in sight. All of a sudden, while still talking to Lana, a thunderous boom sounded, and a deluge of rain ushered streams of water onto my garden, and I almost audibly heard a voice saying, "Eat what is in your garden." Recognizing this voice as being from my heavenly Father, I told Lana that I was getting the answer I needed, and that our drought was over, and my spiritual drought in seeking answers was also over. I could and should eat what was in my garden, which included my chickens and the eggs they so selflessly surrendered to us. After hanging up the phone, I asked God, "Can I eat chocolate?" I heard him simply reply, "Is chocolate in the garden?" I answered, "No, chocolate is not in the garden." Historically, many of my doctors thought a tiny amount of dark chocolate would be permissible, but I knew, with his caring nature, it was not going to be permitted for this season. And truly, it was one of the answers I was looking for.

The following morning, Sunday, August 14, one of our pastors, Jesse Larson, did a sermon titled, "Keep on Keepin' On." He talked about persevering, and if we thought it was time to give up, the answer was no. We must keep on keepin' on. He mentioned that our faith may be tested, and we had to remain faithful to what God has spoken to us and endure without sinking under the pressure. Reflecting over the past few years, when I first had cancer in mere cells which grew to one and then two and possibly three tumors expanding in size, and felt God had told me, "Don't do that surgery," and then, "You will heal naturally; you just weren't slowing down enough to hear me," I felt in my spirit I had to persevere and honor what he told me. The verses he included in his message, scribbled on an envelope I kept in my devotion book, continue to inspire me. "Count it pure joy . . . whenever you face trials of many kinds, because you know that the testing of your faith produces perseverance" (James 1:2–4). "Therefore, my dear brothers and sisters, stand firm. Let nothing move you. Always give yourselves fully to the work of the Lord" (1 Corinthians 15:58). It was as if this could be my work, to write and tell of my story guided by my loving Father to recover and possibly touch someone else along the way to a path of healing. The last verse that struck me was, "You need to persevere so that when you have done the will of God, you will receive what he has promised" (Hebrews 10:36). Jesse concluded by saying that when we are going through a trial or time of testing, we need to change our mindset and stand strong, endure and live our lives with unshakable confidence, and never give up, following the hope God has given us. I was so filled with inspiration after the torrents of rain showered down on my garden, and I felt God had spoken to me about my future healing and how to do what he needed me to do to bring that to fruition. My eyes were welling with tears of hope.

I drove home, and the conversation with God continued. I felt him ask me, "What are the healing colors, Kristi?" I quickly answered, "Blue, green, and purple," and God responded, "Eat those colors." Then he asked, "What are the hot colors?" which I understood as the inflammatory colors, and I answered, "Red, orange, and yellow." He simply answered, "Don't eat those." It was so simple, so easy for me or for anyone to follow. What hit me at a deeper level was the science behind what God had made so easy in this color paradigm, blue versus red. While studying *I Cure Cancer*, the theme of alkaline, no-sugar diets was emphasized over and over again by different doctors. God's instructions divinely aligned with this. The green vegetables were alkaline, and blue and green fruits like kiwi, green apples, and green grapes were lower in sugar or glycemic index. On the contrary, red fruits, such as the tomato, were high in acid, and orange fruits, such as citrus and pineapple, were highly acidic and high in sugar or glycemic index. Also, orange sweet potatoes and carrots, of which I had eaten many during my early attempts at the vegan diet, were high in sugar content. Could it be this simple for me? God was giving me an answer that corresponded with the acid/alkaline and sugar issue and how that related to cancer. To say my mind was blown away would be an understatement.

Running out to my garden, where Tim had planted twenty-three fruit trees to aid in my healing, I noticed that only the green apples were growing, not the red. The red rhubarb, which was highly acidic, was literally shriveled up! I took a picture of it for proof. Our chickens, Daisy, Ruby, Stella, Luna, and Charlotte, were dancing around my feet, pecking at bugs and fruits that had fallen from the trees. I would allow a small portion of meat, eggs, chicken, salmon, and turkey to complement my eating plan. There was an overwhelming confidence that this was it. I found my answers, and I had the clarity to begin to heal. These simple colors in fruits and vegetables, designed by God, would guide me in my healing. I could almost feel the cells in my body begin to heal. They knew just what to do. He then left me with one more message, a silver lining: "When you heal, you can eat fruits and vegetables of all colors of the rainbow."

47

❖

The Finish Line

With excitement in my voice, I called my friend, now Dr. Jessica Yackley, told her my tooth had been yanked and that I had an incredible revelation to share about the "colors of healing," or so I called them. She loved my idea and said, "I would love to support you on this last leg of your journey. We could look at your blood one more time, check the cancer markers, and I could give you our protocol to follow." I hesitated, knowing I had already spent a considerable amount on this natural approach between doctor visits, consultations, and out-of-pocket and copay costs. Her plan was also not going to be cheap. But since she had been supporting me in this phase of my life and was beginning her career with the goal of helping people with cancer, I wanted her to be a part of my medical plan.

At first, there was a prideful response, and I thought to myself, *I have been researching all of this for years, and I don't think I need a protocol or any more supplements or ideas. I know what I need to do.* I called my brother-in-law, Russell Bitter, who was not only family but my prayer partner. I explained my case to him, that it would cost a few thousand dollars more, and I felt I knew enough to proceed. He listened quietly and patiently, then said, "Isn't this the same girl who told you they were missing something, and she was right?" I affirmed that this was the girl. He then said, "What if she has some recommendations you haven't considered that could help you heal? She came along at the right time to inspire you not to give up, right?" While walking on a hill that overlooked the mountains near my home, I told him, "You know, Russell, after all I have done and learned, if I don't follow her protocol and I don't heal, I will always wonder *what if*. I think I have my answer. What is it worth anyway if it can help me heal? It would be worth every penny."

I asked one more friend, Jesse Almanza, if he agreed, since he was also a close friend of mine with great insights when it came to God and his guidance, he agreed that her advice would be worth it and suggested I use the miles on my credit card for a flight to a nice place during this last phase of my journey. He reiterated that if I didn't try the supplements, I may always wonder if they would have helped me get the outcome I wanted.

Jessica wanted to review my most recent labs, and after sending them to her, she noted that I had positive cancer markers in my blood and wanted to make sure this test came back clean after I followed everything she recommended. Her approach was multifaceted, and she wanted to make sure there weren't any negative emotional stressors as I attempted to heal. Interestingly, she noted that my liver wasn't working as efficiently as it could to rid my body of toxins and suggested I do heat and cold contrast baths. Another hot topic came up, that of the coffee enemas I mentioned at the beginning of this book. Wanting me to do these cleansing enemas one to two times a week, for the most part, I was able to fit them into my schedule on weekends. Working five days a week and still struggling with sleep issues, coffee much after 8:00 a.m. would typically wreak havoc on my nights due to its ultra-stimulating effect on my body, so Saturdays it would have to be.

With some hesitation due to the pile of tests and costs associated with each, Jessica requested that I repeat the food sensitivity tests Dr. Mulkey had completed two years prior. Since Dr. Moss in San Diego had said that people like me with autoimmune dysfunction could develop new allergies, as well as allergies to things they ate rather frequently, instinctively, I knew it would be prudent to bite the bullet and the cost and do this test. Shockingly, I learned that I had a sensitivity to cauliflower and to coconut—who would have thought? It was not surprising that when I felt divinely inspired that night, when it was raining on my garden, to eat what was in the garden and only green, blue, and purple foods, cauliflower and coconut, which are white, were not on my list.

Supplements that she suggested were Milk Thistle, also recommended by Dr. Stacy Mulkey, mostly for liver cleansing and immune support. Jessica highly recommended I take several mushroom supplements, and I recall Dr. Mulkey had likewise, but honestly, with the number of supplements suggested, I had not researched mushrooms and wasn't aware of their powerful properties, neglecting to take them religiously after briefly using them at the onset. Jessica highlighted three that she wanted me to take: Chaga, Reishi, and Turkey Tail mushrooms. After going on a walk later that day, and noticing random mushrooms lining the path—something I had not seen in the dry summers we had—I was struck again that I was to eat foods in my environment, and here they were, telling me to take the plunge. We had experienced a very wet winter, with several storms leaving behind two feet of snow at a time, and thus the mushrooms were able to grow in this moist climate. I took both the Turkey Tail and Chaga mushroom supplements in the morning and evening, and the Reishi at night. Researching why I should take these and why Dr. Stacy had recommended them, I was reminded that they cause apoptosis, simply known as cell death, in cancer cells, and could help my body get rid of these abnormal cells. No wonder they both suggested I use them in my protocol. Jessica was concerned that I was not getting enough sleep, a crucial part of our restoration process at night. This was something I had struggled with since I was a child, and she suggested liquid California Poppy for this. Does anyone recall the colorful orange poppies that made the lion, the tin man, the scarecrow, and Dorothy sleep on their way to Oz? Well, this plant is an opioid derivative and definitely made me sleepy! Did it result in sleep? Not always, but I do believe it helped me get there eventually. I also took several ounces of Aloe Vera juice three times a day, good for the intestinal lining.

Steadfast in my ideas for my diet regimen that would be more strict than Jessica recommended, I would implement what she and Dr. Mulkey recommended and begin in mid-August. Both would have permitted me to eat quinoa or gluten-free grains, but I felt I was to restrict these unless I felt my body needed energy, perhaps one to two times a week. In addition, both clinicians would have allowed me to daily enjoy one or two one-inch squares of dark chocolate with no sugar, but since I had already heard a strong voice telling me chocolate chips or squares were not "in the garden," and I had an attachment to it that was a bit too strong, I knew that would be off-limits for the next few months. I felt ready to take a leap of faith, to believe I could heal, and approached my eating plan with gratefulness rather than resentment. A feeling of hope and confidence enveloped me for this phase of the journey. I almost couldn't wait to begin.

48

Healing Waters

D r. Jessica wanted me to do contrast baths weekly if possible, and she had in mind jacuzzis and saunas and cold showers. However, she was just as excited as I was when it struck us that I lived and worked near Pagosa Springs in Colorado. When I first moved to this area with cancer, I had no idea that Pagosa had hot mineral springs, built-in natural jacuzzis. Not only this, but it was next to a winding river fed by melting snow from the Wolf Creek mountains nearby, which would serve as a perfect ice bath. With summertime still in full swing, I could leave work and take a soak in the hot springs and then contrast with a plunge in the frigid San Juan River.

On one particular warm, summer day, and my first opportunity to try the natural contrast baths, I gingerly tiptoed into the "lobster pot," situated right next to the river and at a simmering 104 degrees! I recall that she wanted me to do at least three exchanges of the hot and cold, and try to endure each for several minutes. After thirty seconds in the pot, I was not sure I would be able to withstand the heat, but my body relaxed and I felt sweat beading on my forehead. Honestly, I could have done without the sulfurous smell that emanated from the water, but thankfully, the malodorous vapors were lessened by the breeze and the rapid river a few feet away. Next, I made my way down a few steps onto slippery rocks with a green mossy coating, trying to avoid a fall. Not one to jump in, I inched into the water, getting deeper and, finding an alcove where the rapids weren't flowing, attempted to relax and take slow breaths as I lowered myself until my head was just above the surface. Once I settled into a slow, rhythmic breathing technique, my lungs felt exhilarated, and my muscles celebrated this cold feeling, if even for a short time. With my eyes closed, I imagined the inflammation in my body disappearing, and thanked God that I resided so close to the hot springs and river that surely were helping every inch of my body. Realizing I didn't really take enough time away from work to enjoy this simple pleasure so close to home, I hoped I would take this lesson with me and slow down enough to soak in all that nature had to offer.

After repeating this several times, I prepared for one more cycle in the exhilarating waters. With each set, I had serendipitously met people who were also aware of the benefits of the contrasting waters. They, too, were trying to either reduce inflammation or calm their muscles after a tough hike or mountain bike ride. I also met a few guys who were on an Outward Bound retreat for delinquent youth from the city. They needed the stress relief after handling troubled teens for a few days in the mountains, even though they said the majestic setting quelled many of the negative behaviors. Interesting how nature had a way of doing more than most rehab centers could claim to do in their lives, let alone with everyday people like me.

During my last immersion in the icy cold river, this time making my way beyond the still waters of the alcove, wading into the flowing rapids, and sinking my body into the cool waters, the verse from the most familiar Psalm 23 came to me: "The Lord is my shepherd . . . he leads me beside quiet waters, he refreshes my soul." Surely he was my good shepherd, and surely he was restoring my soul.

Adhering to all her instructions, I also enjoyed saunas at Namaste as often as I could and learned to sit still as sweat poured out of my skin, down my forehead, on my chest, and onto my legs. This was also a lesson in being still, as the sessions lasted nearly half an hour. Not being used to sitting still for long periods of time without reading material, I coined a new phrase for myself, "intentional stillness," while allowing my body temperature to rise and release toxins that I never imagined were there. This stillness in the saunas and the contrast baths in the hot and cold river waters were practices I recommend to "busy" types like me, and they were ones I hope to adopt, with or without the heat or cold surrounding me.

49

✿

Food as Medicine

The remainder of the summer, I welcomed the new eating regimen into my daily routine. Julie encouraged me to be 100 percent compliant, make no excuses, and commit to it with every ounce of my being. Her encouragement and her belief that "we are what we eat" meant so much to me. Needing to prepare some foods ahead of time since I was still working, I used my time wisely and did some juicing, baked purple beets, and sautéed all types of greens so I could comply with this plan every week. Taking the recommendation of Christine and Theo, who I spoke with on the phone in the early days of my cancer diagnosis, I watched the ten-part series by Chris Wark for the second time to glean every ounce of information I could from a man who had stage III colon cancer at age twenty-six and, after colon surgery, used nutrition and natural strategies to restore his health.[21]

The priceless nuggets of information that I gleaned from Chris in his video series were to eat what God created naturally, including as many vegetables and fruits as possible. I recall he felt comfortable eating a

---

[21] Chris Wark, "Square One: Healing Cancer Coaching Series," https://sq1.chrisbeat-cancer.com/module119714539.

specific salad every day with homemade dressing, and he continued to eat this daily, partly out of habit, and partly knowing it was rich in nutrients that could help heal his colon. He recommended avoiding processed food, charred or barbecued foods, foods made with artificial colors, and meat for the most part, unless organic and unless feeling low on energy. He also suggested that those watching pay attention to their mental, emotional, behavioral, and spiritual condition, noting that stress was often linked to cancer.[22]

A close friend from San Diego, Parth Domke, had gifted me a precious, well-made juicer she said she was not putting to good use, and I used this diligently during this phase. It wasn't easy to clean, and I can understand why many buy them with good intentions and leave them in their kitchen cabinets unused, but I was truly on a mission. Using a recipe from Ian Jacklin's book, *I Cure Cancer*,[23] I made my green apple, asparagus, and ginger concoction every weekend and on days when I had the privilege of not working (recipe included in the appendix). I was grateful to Parth for giving me this tool I believe assisted in restoring health to my suffering cells. If plagued by cancer of any type, knowing that cancer is a disease of inflammation and immune dysfunction, consider researching juicing recipes. They have helped many on their healing journey, assisting the immune cells in the body to revive and rid the body of inflammation. Who knows, perhaps it could help give you the energy you were looking for or assist in eliminating toxins in your body. I figured it couldn't hurt, so I used the heck out of this tool in my cancer battle. And have I mentioned that eating this way completely reset and restored my bowel regularity? When eating poorly, ingesting mostly breads and pastas in my twenties, I might only go to the bathroom every two to three days, but on this eating plan, I had regular bowel movements every day, if not after every meal,

---

[22] Wark, "Square One."

[23] Jacklin, *I Cure Cancer*, 22.

three times a day. Headaches, well, they were completely gone—a thing of my past!

Eating clean actually inspired me, and I decided to believe that I was going to recover from this disease without needing surgery. When any doubts or negative thoughts crept in, I held onto something my friend Jerome Stewart taught me: that acting and believing with intention that something was going to happen could bring it to fruition. This process could be called "mind over matter" or compared to "the power of positive thinking," coined by author Norman Vincent Peale in the early 1950s, but I decided that the food I put in my body would be my medicine, and I dove in fully to this plan. Only time would tell.

50

Restoration in Paradise

My sister Julie encouraged me to take some time away, commenting that I hadn't had a true vacation in far too long. We had been given an unexpected gift from our cousin that prior year, and she and Tatiana and then later she, my mom, Aunt Betsy, and cousin Hallee had already been recipients of this treasure, and she thought I should be the next to enjoy what she called an incredible experience. My second cousin, Bruce Dorsey, who lived on the island of Maui, had texted us both in 2020 and asked us if we would be available to do, of all things, a favor for him. He asked if we could come to his home in Hawaii for ten days or more and babysit his outdoor cat, Monster, while he was on a trip to visit his parents in California. Yes, his outdoor cat. Julie and I joked that this was the perfect gig and that we needed to rotate whenever he asked, so no other islander was able to get in on this magical deal. As part of the arrangement, we not only had home accommodations minutes from the beach, but also had access to his truck and could bring up to four people total. Truly yearning to go, but needing to pay for medical costs, I could not afford to go up until this point.

So when Bruce sent a message to both of us in August of 2022, Julie called me right away and said, "Kristi, I will be just completing my move to Austin, and soccer will be in full gear for Damiano, so I hope you can go this time. You and Mom can enjoy the island. This is just what you need right now in your healing." After twisting my mom's arm for a nanosecond, we were in and let Bruce know, per his request, we'd be able to come in mid-September for eleven days! The excitement was mounting as I made work arrangements for other therapists to fill in the gaps while I was gone, and began dreaming of island life, even if for a short time.

On the plane ride there, I was seated next to a beautiful young woman with stunning auburn hair named Rachel Kunde, who wore a necklace bearing a cross, and we began to talk about her college experience and her move to San Francisco for work, after living in Tennessee. We had so many things in common and never ran out of topics to discuss. The first was that she was homeschooled for a season, as was my son. Another area of familiarity for both of us was our lifelong battles with immune issues. Since this was a topic I was well-versed in and had dealt with painstakingly with my own body, and Lukas's as well, we discussed our victories, discoveries, and our current strategies for optimal health. Due to her pure nature, I divulged that I was currently trying to fight cancer naturally, and she asked me to keep her updated and let her know what the results were of my next test, a few months after this Hawaii trip. She offered to pray for me, and with that, I felt healing begin before I set foot on the island.

Soon, she would be reuniting with a lifelong friend who had just ended a difficult relationship and needed some time on the island to gain a new perspective and emotional healing. Later, she talked about the favorite places she frequented when she came to Maui and mentioned she was going straight from the airport to the Lahaina Fish Market and suggested we go to its sister restaurant, the Paia Fish Market, closer to where we would be staying. Although she invited my mom and me to join her in Lahaina, and we touched base and attempted to meet while there, we both went our separate ways, but we have stayed in touch to this day. A feeling blossomed inside of me, talking to her, that this trip was destined to be one of recovery, with a calm sensation spreading from my head to my toes.

After Bruce picked us up from the airport in his white truck with old-school windows that rolled down manually, he took us to The Mill House restaurant, set amongst the heavy metal equipment from a historic sugar mill near his home in Kahului. Birds swooned over the majestic trees they lived in and crooned as the sun began to set, singing a goodnight lullaby before night settled in. Bruce questioned my meal, wondering why I didn't want to order more than asparagus and salmon, and didn't want any bread or starchy foods. Explaining to him that I was trying to beat cancer the natural way, and stating, "You may think I'm crazy, but I am giving this one last shot." Being a pathologist at a nearby hospital in Kahului, he responded, "I don't think you are crazy, even if I might not advise this if I looked at your medical information." With concern in his tone and in his facial expression, he asked me to send my pathology report to him and said that, although it might not be what he recommended, he agreed that my meal choice was a healthy one and asked me to please keep him informed of any further tests.

Since sleep was not one of my natural gifts, I hoped that I would get good rest on this vacation. Earlier that day, my mom and I had to wake up at "zero dark 30" and drive over three hours to the airport in Albuquerque to get here, so my body was wiped out and ready for bed close to 7:30, and I fell asleep without thinking or blinking my eyelids twice. Something rare happened that first morning—I woke up feeling rested. This has only happened to me a handful of times in my life, so I was already ecstatic. Meeting Bruce in his kitchen, way before my mom would wake up, he gave me the "lay of the land" in his home and neighborhood, sharing gate codes and such for my daily morning walks through a lush landscape sprinkled with plumeria trees, whose fragrant aroma was a welcome symbol and "smell of healing" to everyone on the island. My first such walk around his cul-de-sac included a palm tree that announced the creativity of a Creator, with an arc of palms that I could liken to a Native American Indian headdress.

During my first venture to a beach known for some of the best windsurfing in the world near Kahului, with surfers parading their colorful sails as they soared into the air and then plunged into the powerful surf, I was sitting on a beach towel while my mom rested in a lounge chair, and I couldn't help but notice the annoying dry patch of skin that had an eczema-type appearance on the top of my right foot near my ankle. It had been there for several years and persisted through all of my diet changes. My instincts told me to keep an eye on it. Deciding to go on a solo walk, I happened upon the most incredible prehistoric creatures I had ever witnessed—giant sea turtles! There were a plethora of them, and capturing a glimpse of them instantly left me with a feeling of awe. After all, they were ancient reptiles that came before the dinosaurs and also before the formation of the Hawaiian island on whose shores they sunbathed. Tingling coursed through my body, and again, this moment in time marked a feeling of rejuvenation in me. Since my mom had a hip that was accidentally botched during her hip replacement surgery and couldn't walk all the way to see them, I insisted that we get in the truck and drive to another point where she would have a shorter walk to witness them for herself, and she too was able to share in the sacred experience of viewing a live sea turtle.

We planned to travel to the tip of Kapalua, but before doing so, stopped off in the quaint town of Lahaina for breakfast overlooking the ocean, after which we visited the historic banyan tree, which I learned was a gift planted in 1873 from missionaries from India to commemorate the fifty-year anniversary of the first American Protestant mission. Standing underneath its broad canopy and surrounded by sixteen tree trunks, again I felt as if I were standing on holy ground, as such a tree defies reason. After meandering into art galleries and tourist shops with trinkets and refrigerator magnets and keychains galore, we ventured out on the pinnacle of Kapalua. After hiking down a trail that led to a rock formation that resembled the tail and body of a Stegosaurus, my mom and I saw whales breaching their bodies into midair, spouting their breath that collided with the air, creating another moment of awe. Not realizing that this would be one of the last times to see the tree before the horrific fires swept through and nearly destroyed it in 2023, I reflect with gratitude for this experience.

Rather than driving down the entire road to Hana, which many say is one of the most winding and beautiful roads on the planet, we opted for a shorter version with a trip to the Garden of Eden, gardens created by an Australian gardener that were simply, purely, and divinely inspired. The plants, although not native to the island, created angelic sounds heard by the rattling of bamboo, and by the whistling in the wind of birds of paradise, and waterfalls that made one feel as if they had died and gone to the heavens.

Finally, we meandered through lavender fields in the high country where we saw plants that were "Dr. Seussical" and brought laughter and joy to my spirit just standing in their presence. To say this vacation was surreal would be an understatement. With each meal of greens and meat, with handfuls of lush kiwi or blue or purple berries, I could feel my mind, body, and spirit healing.

Monster, a female tabby, developed an affinity toward me. Formerly a stray cat whom Bruce had empathy toward and fed and kept outside at the beginning of their relationship, she now meandered her way in and out of his home as she saw fit. She learned on the first morning of our cat-sitting duties that her cry—more like a deep moan—and thus the name Monster, did not rouse my mom. So she approached me instead every morning around 4:00 to 5:00 a.m., begging not to be touched or comforted, but to be fed a snack or a treat. A sucker for pets, I could not resist. Later, learning that she never did this to Bruce, I realized that Monster had my number and had full control over me. Giving in to her every time—mostly because I wanted to get back to sleep and the treats put an end to that cry—I prepared her smelly, wet, cat food, gave her one or two treats, and fell back to sleep only to be awakened by the natural alarm clock—the song of the mourning doves that were surely prolific in that area. After I got a cup of green tea, I would sit outside next to Monster, who was curled inside a cardboard box that Bruce had crafted for her with a dome-shaped opening. Her cat box rested on a chair at the same table where I sipped my tea and we ushered in each new day together. As I listened to her gentle purring sound and gazed at the clouds that hung over the nearby mountains, I knew Monster and I were a match made in heaven.

On the first Sunday of our trip, my mom and I agreed that we wanted to find an island church to experience the spiritual culture of the native islanders. After googling several churches, I found one that was nearby, and we headed out, giving ourselves ample time to get to our destination before the service began. Approaching the church using phone navigation, I quickly realized we were at a dead-end spot, and the building advertised on the internet looked as if it had been deserted for decades and as if it were from a war-torn region, abandoned and dilapidated. Thank goodness we had our phones and time to spare, so we looked for location number two. Arriving there, we both sensed that perhaps it was too quaint and had a vibe as if to say, we appreciate your interest, but if you are not from here, we would rather you go elsewhere. Also, since there was only one car in the parking lot and the service was about to begin, we didn't really feel we needed to be the only people listening to the poor minister. Maybe the lack of parishioners was a sign he wasn't worth listening to after all. So we looked up our third church, and on the way there, we passed a church with three large crosses that reached into the sky, and we figured even though it wasn't in our Google search, our time was ticking, and we wanted to be at some church on time. As we walked up the stairs to the chapel, we were greeted by people who appeared to be locals or natives of the island, sprinkled with a few visitors and a handful of "haoles" or non-natives like us.

The service was divine. A choir of gospel singers with drums and guitars heralding in songs of worship brought tears to my eyes. The sermon was related to the power of God doing greater things than we imagined—something that resonated with me especially during this time—and we met someone behind us who touched me and reminded me of why I was trying to heal naturally. The visitor we met was a woman who had ovarian cancer that was quite advanced, and when they removed many lymph nodes after her surgery, she gained upwards of forty pounds in her legs. Her doctor would not listen to her or address her concerns about this weight gain, and she suffered for years, until finally she talked to him about it, and she mentioned that she had never been this heavy. He assumed she was obese beforehand, yet this was far from the truth. A physical therapist she went to for leg pain mentioned that she had lymphedema and that with treatment and compression stockings, she could improve and push some of the fluid out of her legs. She was able to successfully lose upwards of thirty pounds of water weight once the therapist pointed her in the right direction, and although she still needed to wear the compression stockings for life, she at least wasn't lugging thirty extra pounds of water weight on her body. Lymphedema post-mastectomy was something I was well aware of and something I wanted to avoid. Remembering the vapid and unempathetic words of my female surgeon who called me "one of those" for not wanting to "let go" of my breast by mastectomy was one of the reasons I was right here in this place, trying to heal naturally, so that my right arm, which I used to treat my patients, would not be swollen like a section of balloon art at the county fair. Giving the woman my hopes for a continued cancer-free life, unburdened by unnecessary lymph fluid, I was surprised by the next part of the church service.

The pastor announced toward the end that anyone who wanted prayer for healing could come forward. This was not something I was accustomed to, although it was more familiar at my country church in Colorado. Without hesitation, I went forward, and a young Polynesian man named Isaiah placed oil on my forehead as it says to do in the Bible. I was familiar with this verse since a woman at my church named Laurel Larson had created a little booklet with every verse in the Bible that included the word "healing." She shared it with me, and I had been meditating on these verses ever since I moved back to Colorado. After sharing with Isaiah that I had breast cancer, and two maybe three cancerous tumors, he prayed for me, also mentioning words from this passage, "Is anyone among you sick? Let them call the elders of the church to pray over them and anoint them with oil in the name of the Lord. And the prayer offered in faith will make the sick person well; the Lord will raise them up" (James 5:14–15). Literally, it was as if energy coursed through my body, and I felt inspired, with a knowing that healing was coming. Tears welled up in my eyes, and I returned to my seat, giving my mom a long hug as tears streamed down my cheeks and I whispered to her that I felt the answer to my prayers was happening before me. Although this church was not on the list of ones I found on my Google search, and we went on a goose chase to find it, I believe it was exactly the one we were supposed to find that day.

My mom and I made one final trip to the beaches of Kahului, where I saw a few women soaking their feet in the water, and I felt drawn to speak with one of their friends who remained behind in the sand closer to the trees lining the shore. Her name was Elizabeth Paravicini, and I learned she ran a camp for underprivileged children in Studio City, California. She had just completed this arduous but fulfilling work and was taking time away on vacation with friends who helped her realize her vision to help the children discover their gifts in the realm of art. She was and is a true inspiration, and we talked of how she felt directed by God to establish this organization and follow her calling, which could inspire children in the field for years to come. We shared how we both felt called to help children in need and encouraged each other in our work and to never stop listening to what God had asked us to do. I believe it was no accident that I met this woman at this time, and I exchanged information with her in case I could ever help to support her cause.

My mom and I spent our last night before leaving the island enjoying

Thai food from a local vendor, and got a cab driver to take us to the airport early the next morning. While walking in the humid air toward the plane with moisture soaking into my skin, I knew this trip to help my cousin Bruce babysit his outdoor cat was more than that. It was a trip to an island where I could take time away from work, time to slow down and eat the food my body needed, and to embrace healing in my mind, body, and spirit. As I boarded the plane, I said, "Aloha," to the people I met, to the majestic island, and to the Creator who formed this wondrous place, certainly with love in His heart.

51

Happy Ninetieth, Papa!

As fall continued, I conspired with my family members to throw a surprise party for my dad for his ninetieth birthday. Orchestrating with Julie to ensure that her husband, Nicola, and kids, Tatiana and Damiano, could be there, we picked the eighth, a few days before his October 11 birthday, and called a few people from out of state to make sure they were free to join us for the celebration. Our cousin, Lesley Mueller—who was one of his biggest fans—was planning on coming until it coincided with plans with her newborn grandson, certainly something we understood. Erica Viviani and Jesse Almanza, also friends with my dad, planned to fly to Durango for the event and said they were here to view the spectacular fall colors that the Aspen trees delivered every year. Kim Weber planned to drive seven hours, also to see the glowing Aspens. My dad fell hook, line, and sinker for all the reasons for being here.

When our family lived in San Diego, Erica and another of my friends, Kim, would come to our house for a visit, and Kim would bring treats such as chocolate chip cookies or brownies. My dad would joke with Kim that next time she came, she should bring a pineapple upside-down cake. She figured we could throw him off to our surprise if she baked a pineapple upside-down cake for an early birthday celebration, and we gave it to him on Friday, the day before the party. She arrived at my home, maraschino cherries and all, and we surprised him with the cake to his utter delight. The smile on his face was something to behold!

Jesse insisted on treating my dad to all of the desserts we would get for the party, including a carrot cake, cupcakes, and chocolate chip cookies. Our family would supply the main course with a spread of lasagna and salad. We made an excuse that he was coming to a church dinner with some of our church friends, Ron and Cindy Bernard, stating that one of them had a party that he was to come to, and he followed suit. He walked into the sanctuary that we transformed into a party space, and we all hollered, "Surprise!" as he almost collapsed with disbelief. Tears rolled down his face as he hugged Tatiana, Julie, Damiano, and Lukas. He gave huge hugs also to my friends Julie and Steve Waltens. We celebrated for hours and then went outdoors to take photos of the attendees. While standing on the hill, in the distance we saw colors of pink and red so bold in the sky, we weren't sure whether to rejoice or take heed in case a storm was on its way. No sooner did most of the guests leave and we had most of the leftover food and desserts packed in our cars, did the storm of the century begin (the lightning bolts were so severe, we learned the next day at the church service that it had knocked out the sound system). Rain came down in torrents, and those of us still bringing things to the cars were drenched. Honestly, it was refreshing, save for the damage to the church, since our area was always in need of rain. We all were able to honor my father for who he was to all of us and enjoy time together.

I mention this evening also because it was the only night in the four months before my next scan that I checked in with myself and allowed myself to eat whatever we had planned for that night. I didn't restrict myself to spinach and a slice of beef or turkey, but ate a huge piece of lasagna and a sizable slice of carrot cake, and even half a chocolate chip cookie. The next morning, I will admit I did feel a little sick to my stomach and also had puffiness under my eyes, indicators of the inflammatory response my body had to these foods, but I enjoyed every bite I took. In my mind, I made sure I believed this one evening of indulgence would not affect my desired outcome. This decision was also bolstered by the French man I spoke of from New York City, with stage three colon cancer that ate "clean" every day for four months, except for those special days between Christmas and New Year's Eve when his mom, a French pastry chef, made croissants, danishes, and treats that he ate and enjoyed. His result was that he was still cancer-free. My hopes mirrored his, and the countdown to test time was upon me. Those who surrounded me at my dad's celebration, Erica, Julie, Jesse, and others, all encouraged me to enjoy myself that day, and prayed for me as test time drew close.

52

The Long-Awaited Answer

November 4, 2022, arrived, and that morning, I could barely take a full breath. After reading a verse or two from a book of inspirational readings, I literally made my way over the river and through the woods to Dr. Chris's house. He met me at his side door with enthusiasm and said, "Are you ready for the results?" With confidence, I said, "I can barely wait!"

First, he had me hold the metal wand in my left hand, and he placed a metal probe into acupuncture points as he looked at the levels on the frequency machine. During the previous test, it showed my right breast to be "unhealthy," with the scan only measuring a number "ten" on the machine, while my left breast and other areas of my body measured a "forty," which was considered healthy. As suspected with my left hand, the dial on the meter continued to climb past the number ten to twenty, thirty, and rested on forty. This was the first good measurement. He then repeated the test with my right hand on my right breast, and again, where the measurement had rested on the dreaded number "ten" months earlier, it now rose to forty! Asking me to take my shoes and socks off, he also tested areas on my feet. Looking down at my right ankle, I surprisingly noticed that the annoying and persistent dry patch of skin was gone. Could it be that my diet changes and my body's improved systemic health had improved the skin on my foot? I could only guess that it had. Next, he confidently said, "With that darn tooth removed, the infection gone, and your body restored, I feel the next test will also confirm that you are cancer-free!"

We both took deep breaths as he asked me to place my hand on a metal device shaped like the outline of the palm of a hand, and he hooked me up to the frequency machine, also used in emergency rooms for diagnostic purposes in Europe. After the machine evaluated my body on many levels I don't understand, it made a computer printout. Before the tooth extraction six months earlier when I was tested, the information stated I had mammary or ductal carcinoma and also odontoid sepsis, or dental infection. This time, these two issues no longer existed. I was infection-free and cancer-free!

Dr. Chris looked me in the eye and said, "Do not speak the word cancer into your body anymore. It is gone, and you don't want to ask it to return." My phone rang, and he saw that it was my son, Lukas. Being familiar with him, he said, "You have to pick up the call and tell him." Answering just in time before he hung up, I said, "Lukas, I just found out my cancer is gone!" He said with excitement, "Mom, I didn't even know you were getting tested today. That is the best news ever!" He told me to call him after the appointment ended, knowing from experience himself with this doctor that the appointments can last several hours. Dr. Chris had also tested Lukas for parasites that plagued him as a child and were identified by name, again on his frequency machine, and later confirmed in bloodwork and other tests. After hanging up the phone, amazed that Lukas would call the instant I got my results, as if he had received a message to call me at that moment, Dr. Chris asked me to go to the treatment room and relax. Before doing that, he said, "I am going to place a laser-type device over your chest. You are not wearing a bra with metal in it, are you?" Perplexed, I answered, "I do have a bra with an underwire in it." With exasperation in his tone, he almost yelled, "You have to remove that. I will leave the room and make sure to take that off before your treatment." Remembering the advice from mine and Lukas's health coach from San Diego, Monica Pelle, who told me not to wear an underwire bra as it could restrict normal lymph flow, after the doctor stepped out, I removed the bra, never to wear one again! He additionally explained that no research had been done as to whether or not the wire could act as a conduit from cell phone energy to exchange unhealthy frequencies to our bodies or breasts. He and Monica had me convinced that it would be better to have sagging breasts in my clothes than have frequencies of energy running through them or restricted flow of lymph in my breast area.

Now, with my chest area free from any wire and with a laser machine covering me, I took deep breaths as tears flooded out of me. In the tiny "treatment hut" beside his home, all the emotions I had experienced in the past nine years since the first day of my cancer diagnosis—when the doctor who had saved my life from my ovarian vein rupturing gave me the hard and honest news that I had ductal carcinoma—poured out of me and onto my chest. The water now was cleansing. Tears I had cried in fear with those first words, "You have cancer," were now tears of relief and joy, streaming with a new message and a new voice, "I am cancer-free!" I had to repeat it to myself several times for the truth to sink in.

The anxiety that kept me up at times at night, dreading the thought of a mastectomy and the possible pain, infection, or after-effects of lymphedema, all welled up and spewed out of me. As I lay on that treatment table, with verses from the Bible visible on the walls of the cabin—placed there purpose-fully by a doctor of Jewish descent—I was overwhelmed with gratitude. A thought came to me, but only fleetingly: "Why did I get to heal? Why did I receive this miracle while others did not?" And the answer came swiftly, "So that you can help others, my child." Another wave of emotions came forth as I wept on that table, sounds of the Pine River from the San Juan Mountains beside his home singing me into a calm state. This battle was over for me.

But another familiar voice came, one I had heard one midnight in my bedroom in October, one year prior, in 2021. That resonating voice I heard when I went to Romania to hold orphans in a town not on the map, and the voice that told me to "find the mother" for Lukas's fourth-grade teacher, had whispered to me then, "You finally slowed down. I have been waiting for you to slow down so I could tell you how to heal. I am going to heal your cancer, and you are going to write about it. It is not for your glory; it is for my glory." Now that same gentle voice said, "You are healed. You can write your story."

When I drove home, responding to Lukas, who had called me and told me to call him back when I was driving home from the doctor, he answered the phone and repeated, "Mom, I didn't know you were getting tested today. I almost can't believe it. I am so happy for you—I am overwhelmed, and it's just unbelievable!" Then I asked him what it was he was going to share with me when he called. He said, "Tim was right. He told me not to listen to anyone in my house who didn't smell that smell I thought might be gas. Remember when Tim and Dr. Stuebe told me to call the gas company? Well, my roommates told me I was imagining things, but they were usually home all day, and when I would come home from work, I noticed a noxious smell. I listened to Tim and called my landlord, but he didn't respond, so I called the gas company, and they came out to the house today (just days after Halloween). The man said he found that propane gas was leaking at dangerous levels out of our water heater, and that had any of us lit even one match in the garage or lit a candle in a pumpkin or something like that, the entire house would have exploded, killing everyone inside. He said if the gas had leaked at any higher level, it could have damaged or killed us since I could smell it inside the home. He found that the landlord didn't have the required carbon monoxide detectors in the house to detect a gas leak. Mom, I'm just so relieved that you are okay, and I am okay too."

I was speechless. If one match had been lit, or if the levels were any higher, my son and his roommates could now be dead. I would have healed but without Lukas in my life. Visions flashed before me in an instant, and again, I was so grateful my story did not end with this disease ending my life, and with my son's life being extinguished. I said, " Lukas, I am so glad you listened to that voice inside."

Since I was approaching Tim's worksite, I told Lukas and he agreed I had to tell him the doctor's findings. I ended the call, stopped by Tim's work in Gem Village, and saw him in the parking lot. Exploding with relief before he could say hello, I said, "My cancer is gone," and he wrapped me in his arms and held me as we soaked in this incredible news.

Next, I nearly ran into my mom's living room and said, "Mom, the cancer is gone. I am healed!" She held me as we wept together, and she repeated, "I knew in my heart this was going to be it! Dr. Chris was going to bring the answers you've been seeking for so many years."

As I write this final chapter, those same tears of gratitude are filling my eyes and falling onto my cheeks. Two and a half years later, still cancer-free, it is time to share this story. I now cry for someone else who is suffering with this disease or another ailment that seems impossible to overcome. This book is not a book proclaiming to heal cancer or heal disease. This is not a book to shame those who have had to make the decision to undergo a mastectomy. If I had an aggressive type of cancer, my path may have been completely different. If someone has prostate cancer or a cancerous brain tumor and the doctors recommend point-specific radiation, I cheer them on for this choice. If they have leukemia or lymphoma at any age and then need chemotherapy, I will pray alongside them as the treatments are delivered. This book is meant to inspire anyone battling an illness, autoimmune or otherwise, to dig deep and ask themselves or their Creator, "What path do you want me to take? How can I best support my body to bring it into the healing it's meant to have?" I do not have all, if any of the answers to so many questions asked, such as, "Why does this person heal and this one does not?" But I know one thing. Ask for help, ask yourself what you feel is needed for healing, and take the step. Have faith and believe it can be so. And that miracle you have been asking for just may come true.

Appendix

Green Apple "Enzyme Juice" Recipe

Juice 1 green Granny Smith apple, ½ cucumber, ½ purple beet, 7 asparagus stalks (cooked), 1 cup broccoli, 2 brussels sprouts, ¼ inch fresh ginger (from the root). Drink within 20 minutes of preparing. The original recipe includes a carrot and pineapple, but due to my inner feelings about not eating orange or yellow fruits, I did not include these.

Foods on my "DO EAT" list

Any green vegetable, including: Spinach, asparagus, broccoli, brussels sprouts, broccoli sprouts, green string beans, kale, celery, artichokes, avocados, purple beets, beet greens, Bok Choy, cabbage, cilantro, cucumber, leeks, garlic, Swiss or rainbow chard (I did not use onions during this phase)

Salt: Sea salt or pink Himalayan salt

Fruits: blueberries, raspberries, blackberries, green apples, plums, kiwi, grapes-green or purple (handful of berries, or one green apple and one serving of each once a day)

Meats: Organic only Salmon, Turkey, Eggs (only 2–3 times a week), red beef, range-free chicken

Grains: gluten-free Ezekiel-type bread (only one slice, 1–2 times a week)

Nuts: pistachios, almonds, cashews, walnuts, pecans (they are all green before they mature and turn brown). Ensure no allergies or sensitivities to these

Teas: green tea, chamomile tea-daily

Butter: Organic – used to sauté my vegetables (I also used avocado oil or olive oil to sauté my vegetables if cooked, and did not use high heat with the olive oil as it breaks down and can release harmful compounds)

Water: Spring water, water using reverse osmosis, or distilled water

Foods on my "DO NOT EAT" list

Anything white, including: bread, white flour, pasta, rice, cereals, potatoes

Legumes: lentils, kidney, red and black beans, garbanzos/chickpeas

Miscellaneous: Corn, chocolate, carob, table salt, tomatoes, any fruit not listed above, alcohol, cocoa, sodas

Dairy: all, except for small amounts of butter, yogurt

Sugars: all, including agave, brown sugar, corn syrup, honey, maple syrup, molasses, sugar substitutes

Peanuts: a commonly allergenic food. I found I was sensitive to this through testing

Soy: a commonly allergenic food, one I was sensitive to

Water: I do not recommend tap water unless it is filtered

Note: (I did not eat cauliflower or coconut as I was tested for food sensitivities after getting my "eat what is in the garden" message and learned I was sensitive to these foods)

Tips for Optimal Sleep

After years of research on insomnia, which I thought I had, I learned ways to optimize my sleep that may help someone else struggling to sleep. My health coach, Monica Pelle, shared some of these suggestions with me, but many I learned along the way. Try any or all ideas.

1. Avoid eating three hours before sleep. Avoid caffeine, including chocolate, for eight hours or more before you intend to sleep, as caffeine can last in the system for up to twelve hours.
2. Avoid computers and TVs (unless using blue light glasses) two hours before sleep.
3. Avoid talking on the phone one hour before sleep. Leave your phone in another room while you sleep if possible.
4. Keep the bedroom at 60–68 degrees.
5. Avoid exercise three hours before bed. The body needs to cool down to sleep.
6. Shower in warm water, and then allow cold water to hit the neck region so the body senses that it is cooling down to prepare for sleep.

7. If you are so exhausted that a nap is required to function, nap for 20–25 minutes and end the nap before 2:00 p.m. if possible, so you don't disturb your circadian rhythm.

8. Keep the bedroom as dark as possible (and keep it free from TVs if possible).

9. Attempt to go to bed at the same time every night. If you sleep in on any day, allow only 30 minutes after your regular rising time to keep your circadian rhythm regular.

10. If you have delayed sleep phase syndrome (DSPS), which is not insomnia—something I believe I have had since birth use these steps to achieve a schedule that other "normal sleepers" have. My system wanted to sleep from 2:00 a.m. to 10:00–11:00 a.m. since I was a small child. If you can fit this schedule into your life, great. If your work or family schedule cannot accommodate this, begin by going to sleep at 2:00 a.m., then reduce that by 15 minutes a night until you achieve success at a time such as 10:00 p.m. As soon as you wake up, go outside and look into the light or sit in front of a light box for 10–15 minutes. Hopefully, this will help you achieve a sleep pattern that works for your lifestyle.

11. Melatonin can assist you in falling asleep, as little as 0.5 to 1 mg. More than this, and it can work in the opposite way. Use a magnesium and calcium supplement two hours before sleep.

12. If you have a paradoxical or opposite reaction to a medicine like Benadryl or Tylenol PM, another medicine with diphenhydramine will cause the same difficulty sleeping.

13. Keep a notebook in your bedroom or nearby, and if any thoughts of things you forgot to do enter your mind, write them down so your mind doesn't fixate on these things.

14. Listen to binaural beats or sleep or theta wave frequencies (if the trickling water and whistling of the wind sounds disturb you, as they do me).

15. Pray or meditate and release all of your thoughts, and ask that your mind be still.

16. Place your feet on the ground, on a rock, or concrete (asphalt is of no benefit) for up to thirty minutes if possible and as weather permits. This "grounding" has been clinically shown to reduce stress, regulate the nervous system, and improve sleep.

End Notes

Gerson, Charlotte. Walker, Morton, DPM The Gerson Therapy. The Proven Nutritional Program for Cancer and Other Illnesses. New York. Kensington Publishing Corp., 2001.

Grigore, Mioara. Cancer, My Love. Platina, CA, USA. St. Heron of Alaska Brotherhood, 2008.

Dr. Haber, Kathryn. Fear Less Love More. What to Do When the Unexpected Happens. Five Daily Choices. Virginia Beach. Koehler books, 2020.

Jacklin, Ian. I Cure Cancer. Learn How to Turn Your Body into a Cancer-Free Zone. USA. Big Distribution, 2019.

McClelland, Jane, PT. How to Starve Cancer without Starving Yourself. United Kingdom. Agenor Publishing, 2018.

Dr. Stengler, Mark, NMD. The Stengler Cancer-Reversing Protocol. Your Personal Guide to the Most Powerful Natural Cancer Therapies. Baltimore. Health Revelations, LLC, 2014.

Wyllie, Carol. Chemo P!ssed Me Off. A Breast Cancer Roadmap: Navigating with Faith, Gratitude, and a Little Bit of Attitude. Dub Press, 2021.

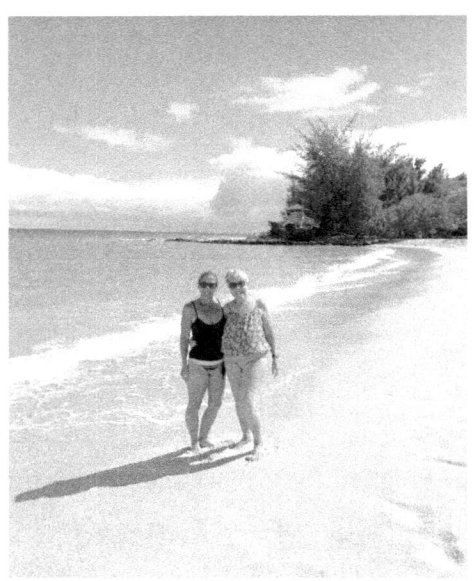

Kristi and her mom Sandi enjoying the beauty of Maui

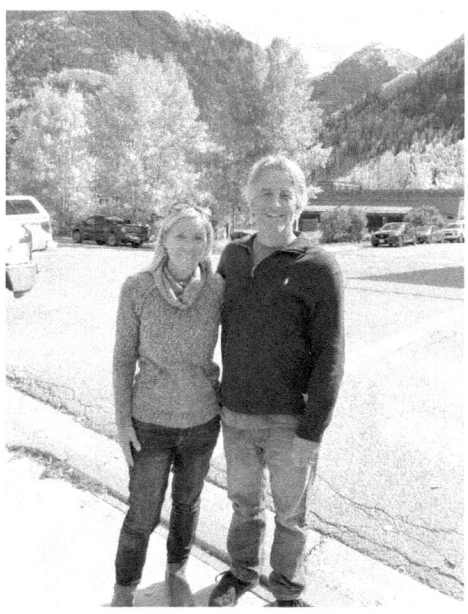

Kristi and her husband Tim on a mountainous
excursion after their move to Colorado

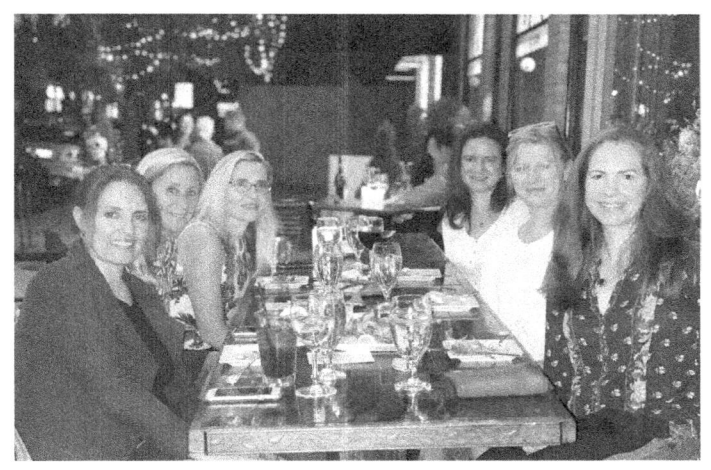

Reunion with Denver coworkers from left and clockwise Nicki Shier, Kristi, Paula Cahill, Lauren Molina, Karin Zimmerman, and Erica Viviani

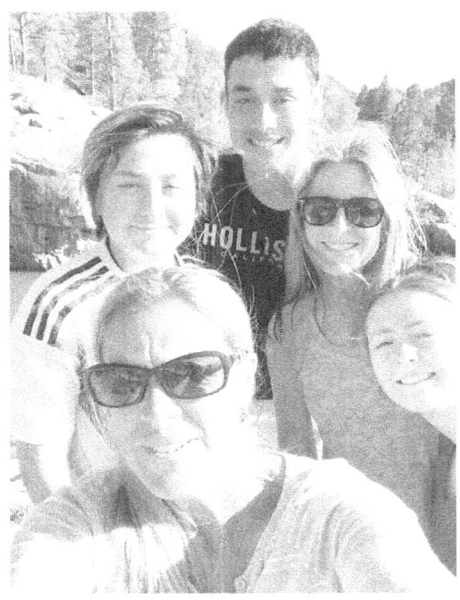

Kristi and her family after her move to the Durango area from center clockwise Kristi, Damiano, Lukas, Julie and Tatiana

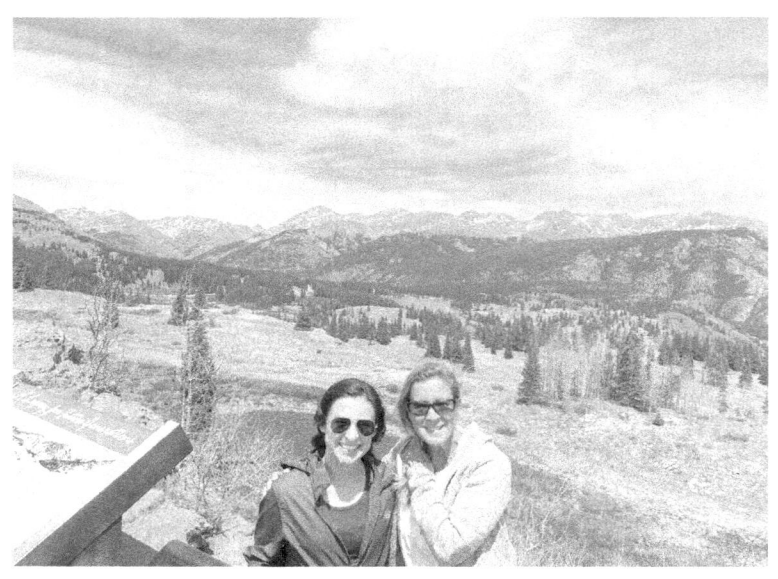

Kristi and her friend and doctor Jessica Yackley
at the top of Molas Pass in Colorado

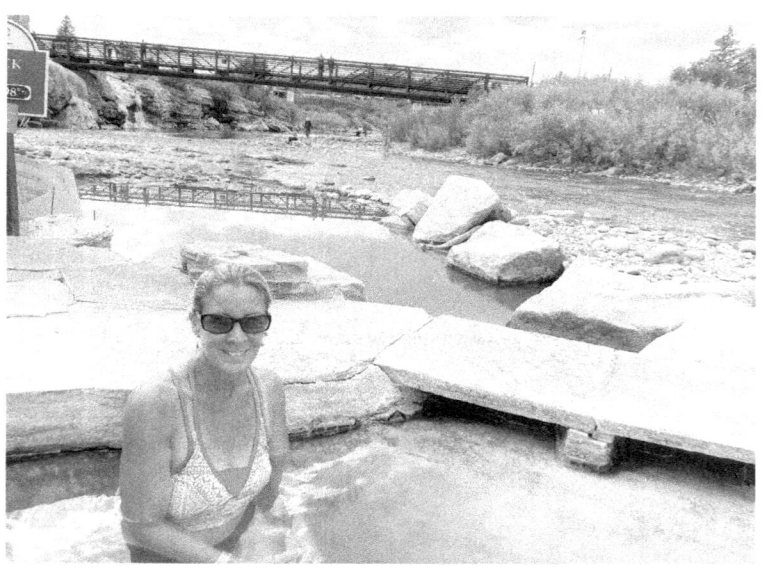

Kristi in the "healing water" of Pagosa Springs, Colorado

About the Author

Kristi Wilkinson spent the first two decades of her life in Pennsylvania and her adult life in the West. She has enjoyed her career as a physical therapist and served as a youth leader, foster parent, and community volunteer. Krist has traveled internationally as a medical volunteer, which led to the miraculous adoption story that inspired her first book, *The Child Who Listens*, and her second book, *The Surrogate Decision*. She resides outside of Durango, Colorado, and works as a PT across the southern region of the state and as a book coach for aspiring writers.

Donations from the book will be given to those challenged with cancer and other health issues.

www.ingramcontent.com/pod-product-compliance
Lightning Source LLC
Chambersburg PA
CBHW071725120626
46550CB00002B/388